Geocoding Health Data

The Use of Geographic Codes in Cancer Prevention and Control, Research, and Practice

Gerard Rushton

Marc P. Armstrong

Josephine Gittler

Barry R. Greene

Claire E. Pavlik

Michele M. West

Dale L. Zimmerman

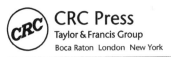

CRC Press

Taylor & Francis Group

Boca Raton London New York

CRC Press is an imprint of the
Taylor & Francis Group, an **informa** business

CRC Press
Taylor & Francis Group
6000 Broken Sound Parkway NW, Suite 300
Boca Raton, FL 33487-2742

First issued in paperback 2019

ISBN-13: 978-0-8493-8419-6 (hbk)
ISBN-13: 978-0-367-38821-8 (pbk)

Library of Congress Cataloging-in-Publication Data

Geocoding health data : the use of geographic codes in cancer prevention and
   control, research, and practice / editors, Gerard Rushton ... [et al.].
      p. ; cm.
   Includes bibliographical references and index.
   ISBN-13: 978-0-8493-8419-6 (hardcover : alk. paper)
   ISBN-10: 0-8493-8419-2 (hardcover : alk. paper)
   1. Cancer--Epidemiology. 2. Cancer--Research--Methodology. 3. Geographic
information systems. I. Rushton, Gerard.
   [DNLM: 1. Neoplasms--prevention & control. 2. Geographic Information
Systems. QZ 200 G342 2008] II. Title.

   RA645.C3G46 2008
   614.5'999--dc22   2007023620

Visit the Taylor & Francis Web site at
http://www.taylorandfrancis.com

and the CRC Press Web site at
http://www.crcpress.com

Table of Contents

Preface

This book had its origin in a project supported by the Centers for Disease Control and Prevention (CDC) to assess issues that arise in the geocoding of cancer incidences and in their subsequent use. In April 2004, we organized a meeting of specialists who had worked with and written about geocodes, mainly in relation to their use in health. Following increasing interest in geocodes and their usefulness in the health community, it became clear to many that a better understanding of them might lead to better realization of their potential in health research and practice. Although this is true in all types of health applications, it is particularly true of cancer, for which specifically where cancers occur is interesting to people trying to understand possible causes of cancer and to others interested in prevention, control, and treatment programs. The many ways in which cancer can be examined in a geographic context can be seen in a series of articles on this subject published on the geography of prostate cancer (Seidman 2006).

This book does not give the last word on most of the issues raised. Geocoding in health is a relatively new subject, and practice is subject to change as new potentials are recognized and new problems encountered. The authors bring experience in a variety of disciplines — geography, health management and policy, law, statistics, and epidemiology. We believe that the issues we examine here will remain important, and the information and evidence provided will help all who work with geocodes in their activities related to health.

We would like to thank colleagues who participated in the specialist meeting in Iowa City, Iowa, in April 2004, and whose ideas and encouragement led to this book: Toshi Abe, Luc Anselin, Randall Bezanson, Robert Borchers, Frank Boscoe, Jim Holt, Sue-Min Lai, Eugene Lengerich, Junlin Liao, Charles Lynch, Mark Monmonier, and Patrick Remington.

We want to thank in particular our project officer from CDC, Tom Richards, for the many leads to interesting developments in geographic information systems and geocoding in health. Several graduate students at the University of Iowa helped us develop these materials. Most appear as coauthors in chapters on which they worked.

REFERENCE

Seidman, C. S. 2006. An introduction to prostate cancer and geographic information systems. *American Journal of Preventive Medicine* 30(2), Supplement, S1–S2.

Editors and Contributors

Toshi Abe
New Jersey Department of Health
  and Senior Services
Trenton, New Jersey

Marc P. Armstrong
The University of Iowa
Iowa City, Iowa

Kirsten M. M. Beyer
The University of Iowa
Iowa City, Iowa

Francis P. Boscoe
New York State Department of Health
Albany, New York

Qiang Cai
The University of Iowa
Iowa City, Iowa

Zunqiu Chen
The University of Iowa
Iowa City, Iowa

Josephine Gittler
The University of Iowa
Iowa City, Iowa

Barry R. Greene
The University of Iowa
Iowa City, Iowa

Claire E. Pavlik
The University of Iowa
Iowa City, Iowa

Gerard Rushton
The University of Iowa
Iowa City, Iowa

Alan F. Schultz
California Department of Health
  Services
Sacramento, California

Geoffrey Smith
The University of Iowa
Iowa City, Iowa

David G. Stinchcomb
The National Cancer Institute
Bethesda, Maryland

Chetan Tiwari
The University of Iowa
Iowa City, Iowa

Lance A. Waller
Rollins School of Public Health
Emory University
Atlanta, Georgia

Michele M. West
The University of Iowa
Iowa City, Iowa

Dale L. Zimmerman
The University of Iowa
Iowa City, Iowa

1 Introduction

Gerard Rushton, Marc P. Armstrong, Josephine Gittler, Barry R. Greene, Claire E. Pavlik, Michele M. West, and Dale L. Zimmerman

CONTENTS

1.1 GEOGRAPHIC INFORMATION SYSTEMS AND DISEASE MAPPING

New methods for recording the locations of disease have permitted new types of disease mapping and new methods to support disease prevention and control activities in public health. From these developments, new understandings of disease risk factors may be found that may lead to new treatment patterns as well as disease prevention and control activities.

In the past, disease patterns were mapped and analyzed primarily at the level of political units, such as states, counties, or census tracts. The same units were used to define health service areas and to measure people's access to service using ratios of people to services available in these rather arbitrary units. Now, however, geographic information systems (GISs) allow a new level of detail and precision, and thus flexibility, regarding geographic location because they enable the "geocoding" of residential addresses to point locations using digital street databases and other types of geospatial data.[1,2] This detailed geography of disease permits the mapping of many types of geographies, such as disease rates in relation to pollution sources. Geographic detail also permits clearer identification of areas of need and for improved health service

1

provision. Balancing the availability of such precise information, however, are concerns about maintaining the privacy and confidentiality of individuals as required by law,[3] as well as securing reliable estimates of disease rates.[4]

1.2   THE SIGNIFICANCE OF GEOCODING METHODS

These new methods for recording location are known as *geocoding methods*. The U.S. Department of Health and Human Services highlighted potential benefits of geocoding in its policy-setting document *Healthy People 2010* (section 23-3):

> The capacity to achieve national goals is related to the ability to target strategies to geographic areas. Extension of geocoding capacities throughout health data systems will facilitate this ability. ...
>
> However, public access to data below the county level is prohibited or severely restricted because of confidentiality and privacy issues.
>
> A major challenge in the coming decade will be to increase public access to GIS information without compromising confidentiality.[5]

With recent disease outbreaks such as SARS (severe acute respiratory syndrome), the anticipation of potential global impacts of bird flu, concerns about bioterrorist attacks, and plans to reduce health disparities, the interest of both public health and governmental officials in the application of GISs to individual-level data has clearly grown. However, to date no book focuses on geocoding health data, including the privacy and confidentiality issues that this presents. Geocoding methods are also significant because increasingly geocodes and methods of spatial interpolation and prediction that use them are used to provide geographic detail in cancer maps that formerly could not be made with any reliability.[6–8]

1.3   SCOPE OF THIS BOOK

This book has two purposes. First, it aims to identify and discuss the many issues that arise when geocodes are made and used in public health research and practice. Second, it aims to show how the findings of research studies that use geocodes, as well as health services programs that use them, need to be based on geocodes of sufficient quality to meet the purposes for which they are used. Most public health professionals, for whom this book is written, are not well versed in the characteristics and availability of geospatial data and in the methods used to link different types of geographical identifiers. This book describes such types of geographical identifiers, how they become formal geocodes, and then how they are used.

This volume uses cancer control and prevention programs to illustrate these ideas, although geocoding can be used for many other health applications because the basic principles of geocoding practice do not vary from one public health application to another. The book focuses on a significant public health problem, cancer, to demonstrate how the availability of geocoding can be used in research and practice to address the provision of prevention and control activities as well as to achieve a better understanding of the distribution of the disease. In particular, it draws on the experience and expertise of cancer registries in North America and incorporates discussion of the cancer data sets they have developed and their application to prevention and control activities. We note the recent growth in the geographic and comprehensive data coverage of the many new state cancer registries in North America. In particular, we address (1) how geocoded residential addresses can be used to examine the spatial patterns of cancer incidence, staging, survival, and mortality and (2) how privacy and confidentiality issues may be addressed by focusing on disclosure limitation methods while simultaneously enabling more accurate and detailed spatial data on disease distributions to be used. The book presents a state-of-the-art discussion based on current developments.

This book also covers the many technical and administrative developments in geographic information science that will affect the future practice of geocoding. Geocoding has been the subject of many reviews.[9–12] A further purpose here is therefore to integrate the findings and conclusions of these reviews.

Because geocodes are used in processing health data, many issues arise in their use. This book describes these issues and discusses implications with respect to the many purposes for which geocodes are used. In addition to the reason that incidences of cancer are increasingly geocoded, we focus on cancer because of the substantial increase in public health activities designed to understand local geographical measures of the burden of cancer and the increase in geographic-based activities to prevent and control cancers. It is now widely recognized that the characteristics of communities and their neighborhoods influence the rates of cancer incidence, staging, survival, and mortality. Also influencing these rates are different levels of access to resources for cancer prevention and control.[13–15] Cancer was chosen as the focus both because of the level of concern regarding its personal and social burdens and to demonstrate how methodological and data improvements can assist in prevention and control activities, including the improvement of health service allocations. The same principles used to geocode cancer are similar to the process for geocoding other health data.

1.3.1 Purpose of Attaching Geocodes to Data

Attaching geocodes to health data and many other types of data to which health data are related has become a basic activity in public health research and practice. Geocoding practices — the steps taken to find geocodes for such data — are changing rapidly as more ways are developed to accomplish the end of attaching geographic identifiers to data. Geocodes have become useful in public health research and practice because they provide linkages between disparate data that contribute to health and disease in populations. Before the word *geocode* was used, geographic linkages between data were typically made for fairly large pieces of geography. In the United States, states and counties were the typical geocodes used, and data were collected for these units.

As concerns over differences in health in populations grew, however, the practice developed of investigating health at the level of the individual and the individual's family. Risk factors for disease were identified as individual behaviors that needed to be changed. More recently, it has become the practice to add to individual-level risk factors the societal and neighborhood factors that also contribute to ill health and to its treatment. Now, we recognize many geographic levels at which forces operate to produce ill health or to bring about its alleviation.

Measurement theories now often leave open to investigation the appropriate geographic level at which these forces operate, and studies are designed to identify these levels for particular diseases. These geographic levels change through time. Geographical differences in infant mortality in the United States 70 years ago, for example, were primarily between the major regions of the country, but today the differences are primarily within each region and frequently within metropolitan counties. The geographic scale at which the appropriate geocode works has changed in this period.

As the geographic scale at which linkages between disparate data were made began to focus on smaller geographic units and as different results began to be found with different spatial units, it became clear that it was important to control the spatial unit of analysis so that the correct spatial scale at which relationships existed could be discovered and presented in ways that could be communicated to others. With that, the science and language of geocoding began. We became interested in the methods and the materials by which geographic identifiers could be attached to data, in ways of communicating to others about methods and materials used, and in discovering which, if any, method produced the most useful results. We also became interested in methods to protect the privacy of individuals because many geocodes are essentially personal identifiers in the same sense that a personal telephone number can usually be linked to a telephone book of such numbers and names; thus, full identification can be found. These developments are illustrated in Figure 1.1; health maps at the bottom of the figure are shown as produced by linking health data to geographic framework data for the area in question.

Figure 1.1 shows the forces that have led to the increased use of geocoding in public health. Three factors are recognized in the figure. First, at the top of the figure are geographic base files that form a framework to which other data can be attached. It is the increased availability and accuracy of these geographic base files that has led to the widespread adoption and use of geocoding methods in public health. Other data are health data, socioeconomic data, or other environmental data with geographic identifiers that can be linked to the geographic base files. At the bottom of the figure are the mapping application programs. All three areas of inputs in this process have developed greatly in the past decade.

1.3.2 Geographic Framework Data

Since 1993, federal, state, and local governments have contributed to the establishment of a digital national spatial data infrastructure.[16] A key element of this effort is geographic framework data, which consist of themes such as cadastral information and transportation networks.[17,18] Such themes are important in the context of this book because they are used to support geocoding. Street networks have been compiled into a national-level database; each link in the network (links are typically defined between intersections) has an associated set of attributes, such as the range of addresses on each side of the street, as well as information about political and administrative jurisdictions to which the street segment belongs. These framework data enable the integration of numerous disparate types of information through the common theme of location. Developments such as GNSS (global navigation satellite system) and digital orthophotography have increased the ability of researchers and data users to locate features of interest with high levels of accuracy. This capability leads to a process, with proper quality control and assurance, through which framework data can be routinely updated to ensure closer correspondence between the

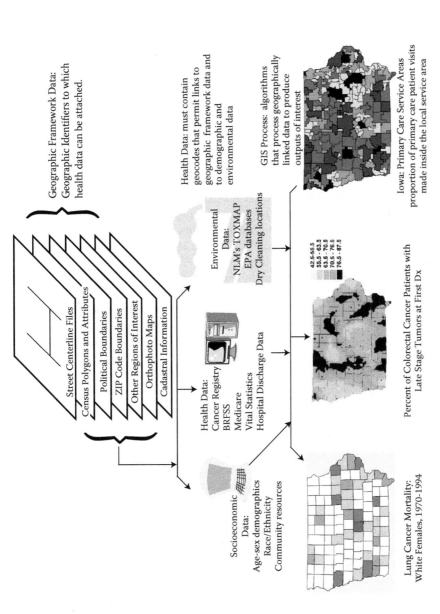

FIGURE 1.1 Factors leading to increased use of geocoding in public health: geographic framework data; geocoded health, demographic, and environmental data; and GIS data-processing algorithms.

administrative records used as geocoding inputs and the digital representations of geography used to assign locations to these records.

1.3.3 PRIVACY CONSIDERATIONS WITH GEOCODED DATA

As noted throughout this book and discussed in detail in chapter 12, certain types of geocodes can be used to identify individuals. Cancer registries, state health departments, or other groups with access to geocoded records of cancer cases are required by law to protect the privacy of individuals, especially when state law mandates that their personal health information be given to these groups. Thus, the benefits that can be gained by analyzing cancer data in its geographical context cannot be gained at the expense of the harm that would occur if ever the privacy of individuals was not adequately protected.

1.3.4 ISSUES WITH THE SPATIAL STATISTICAL ANALYSIS OF GEOCODED DATA

Spatial statistical analyses of geocoded health data offer the possibility of addressing many important public health questions. For example, a spatial statistical analysis can determine whether an apparent cluster of disease cases is too unusual to be reasonably regarded as having occurred by chance alone. Also, if a geographically varying disease risk factor (such as distance to a pollution source) is measured for each individual in the at-risk population, then a statistical analysis can detect and quantify possible associations between the disease and this risk factor.

However, valid spatial analyses of geocoded health data rest on the assumptions that geocodes are complete and correct. Although this may often be sufficiently well satisfied for area-level geocodes such as ZIP codes, for point-level geocodes it is not. In fact, it is common for 10%–30% of subjects' addresses to fail to geocode to a point location, and of those that do, positional errors of hundreds of meters are common. The incompleteness and inaccuracy of geocodes generally have an adverse effect on statistical analyses and can lead, if ignored, to conclusions of dubious value. For example, the power to detect a disease cluster decreases as the magnitudes of positional errors increase, becoming badly degraded when these magnitudes are on the same scale as the cluster size itself. Likewise, the ability to relate disease incidence to a geographically varying risk factor is severely limited if positional errors are commensurate with the scale at which the risk factor operates.

The statistical methodologies of missing data analysis, coarsened data analysis, and measurement error modeling have been brought to bear on the problems of incomplete and incorrect geocoding. These methods properly reckon with geocode incompleteness and positional errors in the detection of clusters and other spatial analyses, thus allowing statistically valid conclusions to be drawn from the data.

1.3.5 GEOGRAPHIC MASKING OF GEOCODED DATA
FOR CONFIDENTIALITY PROTECTION

Although accurate point-level geocodes confer the greatest possible power on spatial statistical analyses, they also may, through a process known as reverse geocoding, make it possible for anyone who obtains the geocodes to determine the address and hence the identities of persons to whom the geocode and its concomitant information correspond. Thus, the release of geocoded data by its owner or custodian to researchers or other users may violate privacy laws or agreements under which the data were originally collected.[19] *Geographic masking* is a process by which highly accurate geocodes are modified to an extent sufficient for the data to be released to users. Ideally, a geographic mask will retain enough spatial accuracy for true clusters, real relationships with risk factors, and the like to be detected with reasonably high power while keeping the risk of individual identity disclosure below an acceptable threshold. Some common geographic masks include affine transformations (e.g., a rigid translation), aggregation to areal units, and random perturbation. In addition to the choice of mask and the level of masking, issues the data custodian must consider include the amount of information about the mask (mask metadata) that should be disclosed to data users and whether multiple masked versions of the data may be safely released to satisfy different analysis objectives among multiple users.

1.3.6 Geocodes as the Basis for Distance Measures

Geocoding is typically a preliminary (but necessary) step to further analysis. After a coordinate or other geocode has been added to a record, it becomes possible to compute geometrical relationships between these records or between them and other locations in the landscape that are represented as points, lines, or areas. Although measures such as dispersion and directional statistics may be performed on geocoded records, a common form of analysis requires the calculation of distances.

There are several ways to find distances from geocodes. In general, distances are computed between points using some metric, or they are computed using a digital representation of a road network. Interpoint distance metrics assume different forms depending on the nature of the study area under consideration. If accurate long (hundreds of kilometers) interpoint distances are required, then it is a good practice to compute distances using latitude and longitude and a spherical distance metric. For shorter distances, projected Cartesian coordinates can be used with relatively high accuracy. These coordinates are then used with formulae that compute Euclidean (so-called crow-fly) distances or rectilinear (Manhattan) distances such as are found in large parts of the central United States and in many large cities. In other cases, an empirical parametric approach may be used. In such cases, a sample of distances is used to estimate a parameter that can be substituted in place of the 2 (Euclidean) or 1 (Manhattan) exponent.

In the previous cases, estimated distances do not take account of the road network and the possible routes that a patient may select to travel to a health facility. If geocoded locations are coordinates located on a road network, such as a TIGER (Topologically Integrated Geographic Encoding and Referencing) line file, and if the road network has been coded with distances (or travel times) between all nodes, then shortest distances from the known location to all other nodes on the network can be computed using a shortest-path algorithm, although there is widespread appreciation of the fact that people will often neither use their nearest health facility nor take the shortest route to the one selected.

If the geocodes are areas such as census tracts, then distances can be computed from their centroids. These distances are rough estimates, but they may be adequate for some purposes. It is important to realize, however, that errors occur when many people are assigned to the centroid of an area. This is known as *spatial aggregation error.*

1.3.7 DISEASE REGISTERS AND GEOCODING ISSUES

In an effort to accelerate, enhance, and focus the national cancer effort in 1971, a committee of experts recommended collecting both cancer incidence and survival data on a continuous basis from the same set of patients. From that recommendation, the Surveillance, Epidemiology, and End Results (SEER) Program of the National Cancer Institute (NCI) was born and was codified in the National Cancer Act of 1971. The SEER Program currently collects and publishes cancer incidence and survival data from population-based cancer registries covering approximately 26% of the U.S. population. The National Program of Cancer Registries (NPCR), established by Congress through the Cancer Registries Amendment Act in 1992 and administered by the Centers for Disease Control and Prevention (CDC), supports central cancer registries in 45 states, the District of Columbia, Puerto Rico, the Republic of Palau, and the U.S. Virgin Islands. These data represent 96% of the U.S. population. Together, NPCR and the SEER Program collect data for the entire U.S. population. For a map detailing NPCR and SEER registries, see http://www.cdc.gov/cancer/npcr/npcrpdfs/0607_npcr_fs.pdf. For a list of other organizations also involved in cancer surveillance, visit http://www.seer.cancer.gov/about/activities.html.

NCI staff work with the North American Association of Central Cancer Registries (NAACCR) to guide all state registries to achieve data content and compatibility acceptable for pooling data and improving national estimates. NAACCR's membership is comprised of 13 central cancer registries in Canada and more than 50 central cancer registries in the United States. NAACCR formed a committee to address the appropriate uses of GISs in cancer registry practice. This GIS committee compiled a report in 2002, *Using Geographic Information Systems Technology in the Collection, Analysis and Presentation of Cancer Registry Data: A Handbook of Basic Practices.*[20] The handbook is a current reflection of how GISs can be applied to cancer registry operations, practices, and even research using cancer registry data.

Central cancer registries in North America routinely collect information on the residential address of each person at the time of diagnosis. Some registries also collect information on a current address for follow-up purposes. The address at time of diagnosis is used by epidemiologists for a variety of purposes, including cancer cluster investigations and for use in assessing cancer patterns for cancer prevention and control activities. Accurately geocoding the address at time of diagnosis is crucial for these activities. Accuracy is based on the match rate (the percentage of cases that are successfully geocoded) as well as the positional accuracy of the geocode (how close the estimated location is to the true location). In this book, we discuss current methods available to ensure the most accurate data possible as well as future improvements that may aid cancer registries.

1.4   CONCLUSIONS: THE AUDIENCE FOR THIS BOOK

This book meets the interests and needs of a public health workforce as well as a large research community that increasingly is expected to address the where as well as the what and the when of cancer mortality, disease, and prevention and control activities. The potential audience also includes health care administrators as well as the public. These constituencies have in common a desire to see geographic detail in spatial patterns of disease and death. They ask for geographic downscaling of the cancer maps they are accustomed to seeing. Unfortunately, only recently has the science of spatial epidemiology become interested in such spatially explicit questions.[8,21–23] Geocoding cancer data with a variety of geographic reference data permits such maps to be made. Theory and methods in geographic information science (GIS) provide the tools to pursue these ends.

REFERENCES

1. Federal Geographic Data Committee National Spatial Data Infrastructure. http://www.fgdc.gov (accessed July 19, 2007).
2. Federal Geographic Data Committee, Data and Services. http://www.fdgc.gov/dataandservices/(accessed July 19, 2007).
3. Centers for Disease Control and Prevention. HIPAA privacy rule and public health. Guidance from CDC and the U.S. Department of Health and Human Services. *MMWR Morb Mortal Wkly Rep* 2003, 52 Suppl, 17, 19–20.
4. Elliott, P.; Wakefield, J. C.; Best, N. G.; Briggs, D. J. *Spatial Epidemiology: Methods and Applications.* Oxford University Press, Oxford, U.K., 2000, p. 465.
5. U.S. Department of Health and Human Services. Public health infrastructure, chapter 23 in *Healthy People 2010.* http://www.healthypeople.gov/Document/HTML/Volume2/23PHI.htm (accessed February 13, 2007).
6. Atkinson, P. M.; Tate, N. J. Spatial scale problems and geostatistical solutions: a review. *Prof Geogr* 2000, 52, 607–23.
7. Kyriakidis, P. C.; Yoo, E. H. Geostatistical prediction and simulation of point values from areal data. *Geogr Anal* 2005, 37, 124–51.
8. Goovaerts, P. Exploring scale-dependent correlations between cancer mortality rates using factorial kriging and population-weighted semivariograms. *Geogr Anal* 2005, 37, 152–182.
9. Rushton, G.; Armstrong, M. P.; Gittler, J.; Greene, B. R.; Pavlik, C. E.; West, M. M.; Zimmerman, D. L. Geocoding in cancer research: a review. *Am J Prev Med* 2006, 30 (2 suppl), S16–24.
10. Goldberg, D. W.; Wilson, J. P.; Knoblock, C. A. From text to geographic coordinates: the current state of geocoding. *URISA J* 2007, 19, 33–46.
11. Krieger, N.; Zierler, S.; Hogan, J. W.; Waterman, P.; Chen, J. T.; Lemieux, K.; Gjelsvik, A. Geocoding and measurement of neighborhood socioeconomic position: A U.S. perspective. In *Neighborhoods and Health*, Kawachi, I.; Berkman, L. F., Eds. Oxford University Press, Oxford, U.K., 2003, pp. 147–78.
12. Yang, D.; Bilaver, L.; Hayes, O.; Goerge, R. Improving geocoding practices: evaluation of geocoding tools. *J Med Syst* 2004, 28, 361–70.
13. Athas, W. F.; Adams-Cameron, M.; Hunt, W. C.; Amir-Fazli, A.; Key, C. R. Travel distance to radiation therapy and receipt of radiotherapy following breast-conserving surgery. *J Natl Cancer Inst* 2000, 92, 269–71.

14. Schroen, A. T.; Brenin, D. R.; Kelly, M. D.; Knaus, W. A.; Slingluff, C. L., Jr. Impact of patient distance to radiation therapy on mastectomy use in early-stage breast cancer patients. *J Clin Oncol* 2005, 23, 7074–80.

15. Nattinger, A. B.; Kneusel, R. T.; Hoffmann, R. G.; Gilligan, M. A. Relationship of distance from a radiotherapy facility and initial breast cancer treatment. *J Natl Cancer Inst* 2001, 93, 1344–46.

16. National Research Council of the National Academy of Sciences. *Toward a Coordinated Spatial Data Infrastructure for the Nation*. National Academy Press, Washington, DC, 1993.

17. Moeller, J. J.; Reichardt, M. E. National, international, and global activities in geospatial science. In *Manual of Geospatial Science and Technology*, Bossler, J., Ed. Taylor and Francis, New York, 2002, pp. 593–607.

18. Warnecke, L.; Decker, D. Geographic information technology in state governments of the United States. In *Manual of Geospatial Science and Technology*, Bossler, J., Ed. Taylor and Francis, New York, 2002, pp. 575–592.

19. Brownstein, J. S.; Cassa, C. A.; Mandl, K. D. No place to hide — reverse identification of patients from published maps. *N Engl J Med* 2006, 355, 1741–1742.

20. Wiggins, L. (Ed.). *Using Geographic Information Systems Technology in the Collection, Analysis, and Presentation of Cancer Registry Data: A Handbook of Basic Practices*. North American Association of Central Cancer Registries, Springfield, IL, October, 2002, 68 pp.

21. Elliott, P.; Wartenberg, D. Spatial epidemiology: current approaches and future challenges. *Environ Health Perspect* 2004, 112, 998–1006.

22. Kelsall, J.; Wakefield, J. Modeling spatial variation in disease risk: a geostatistical approach. *J Am Stat Assoc* 2002, 97, 692–701.

23. Ostfeld, R. S.; Glass, G. E.; Keesing, F. Spatial epidemiology: an emerging (or re-emerging) discipline. *Trends Ecol Evol* 2005, 20, 328.

2 Geocoding Methods, Materials, and First Steps Toward A Geocoding Error Budget

Marc P. Armstrong and Chetan Tiwari

CONTENTS

2.1 INTRODUCTION

Records that contain street addresses are often found in database systems that are used to monitor the health transactions of medical patients. Although addresses can be used by humans to establish locations, computer systems require more explicit representations to produce maps and conduct analyses. *Geocoding* is a process through which records without explicit location identifiers are enhanced by the addition of coordinates or geographic identifiers such as census enumeration units.[1] In its most typical form, geocoding takes records with addresses and assigns a latitude and longitude value (or other geographic identifier) to each. The purpose of this chapter is to describe the materials that are used to support geocoding, to illustrate geocoding methods, and finally to sketch the types of errors often encountered. An awareness of error types is valuable when attempting to ensure that the results of geocoding are accurate. This has implications for quality control and assurance as well as project management.

2.2 MATERIALS

Two types of materials are used during geocoding. The first is a collection of records, often stored in either a relational database or as a flat file, that contain a patient's medical history, record of treatment, or other epidemiological information. For example, a record about a patient with prostate cancer might contain information about his home address at time of first diagnosis, treatment type received, address and name of the treatment facility, and dates of treatment. The second type of material used during geocoding is referred to as a *geographic base file* (GBF). This file supports the establishment of a correspondence between the administrative records and details about the geographic characteristics of a place, such as political jurisdictions, census enumeration areas, and coordinates of features. In the following sections, we describe each type of information and discuss ways to ensure high-quality input and output from geocoding processes.

2.2.1 THE ADDRESS

The address fields contained in the collection of records to be geocoded must be processed by software, and as a consequence, the use of a standardized format will ultimately lead to fewer errors. The Address Standards Working Group

(ASWG) of the Federal Geographic Data Committee has defined four general types of addresses:[2]

- *Thoroughfare:* specifies a location along a linear feature, normally a thoroughfare of some type (e.g., 1225 Rochester Street)
- *Postal:* provides a mechanism for mail delivery to a central place without reference to the residence location of an individual (e.g., PO Box 280, Anytown, IA)
- *Landmark:* specifies a location through reference to a well-known feature (e.g., Madison Square Garden)
- *General:* a mix of the first three classes

The most commonly encountered types in this classification are the first and second. Moreover, addresses in these classes tend to have a general format that can be used to guide expectations about the order in which address elements will appear; such knowledge can also help to reduce errors.

- *Address number element:* This is usually a sequentially sorted integer identifier that provides information about the relative location of an address with respect to the extent of the linear entity described as a street name element. This element may contain fractional values and may have other prefix and postfix information added (e.g., 1234 D).
- *Street name element:* This element is often modified. In its most primitive form, it is simply an unambiguous street name, such as Main Street, but there are a host of modifiers in common use:
  - *Premodifier:* Includes terms such as "Old" or "Great" (e.g., Old Shaker Road).
  - *Predirectional:* Usually refers to a cardinal direction.
  - *Pretype:* A street style is sometimes a modifier (Avenue of the Saints).
  - *Name:* The primary name recognized by local government.
  - *Posttype:* The conventional street style (road, avenue) that is affixed to an address.
  - *Postdirectional:* See Predirectional.
  - *Postmodifier:* Occurs at the end of street address to refine the identification of a thoroughfare.
- *Building, floor, and unit elements:* These are used typically for multiresidential unit structures to identify particular apartments and other forms of dwellings.
- *Larger-area elements:* These elements refer not only to municipal jurisdictions and state names or abbreviations but also to elements such as ZIP codes.
- *USPS (U.S. Postal Service) postal address elements:* Box numbers and other identifiers are included in this element type.

When address information is structured using an expected format, it is possible to parse the input data into the standard set of elements. One such format that is widely adopted is specified by the USPS in its Publication 28, *Postal Addressing Standards*.[3] This standard calls for an address that is comprised of three lines, uses capital letters and USPS standard abbreviations, and omits punctuation except for the hyphen in the ZIP + 4 code:

Recipient line → ROBIN DOUGH
Delivery address line → 1234 E MAINE ST STE 2001
Last line → COLUMBUS OH 54321-0010

In this example, a directional prefix (E) is used along with a secondary unit designator (STE 2001) to identify a location within a multiunit address. The full set of components, used in parsing each address, is as follows: primary address number, predirectional, street name, suffix, postdirectional, secondary address identifier, and secondary address range. It is expected that the city names in the last line will be spelled in their entirety, although the USPS[3] has compiled a list of standardized abbreviations for city names, state names, and street suffixes. For example, the commonly used street suffixes or abbreviations for *boulevard* are contained in the set {BLVD | BOUL | BOULEVARD | BOULV} with the standard (preferred) abbreviation BLVD. The USPS also has a related set of address standards that apply exclusively to the Commonwealth of Puerto Rico because it uses a set of conventions that are inconsistent with those used elsewhere in the United States, apart from the extensive use of Spanish.

2.2.2 DATA ENTRY AND MAINTENANCE

Errors in input data will inevitably decrease the quality of geocoding results. Consequently, steps taken to reduce the introduction of errors, as well as to eliminate them once detected, will ensure that a greater proportion of records is correctly geocoded. One way to achieve high standards is to establish a set of protocols for data collection and entry personnel. These protocols draw on the standard described in the preceding section and fall into three major categories:

• Spelling errors and exceptions
• Abbreviations
• Prefixes and suffixes

Field workers, clerical staff, or data entry personnel can be taught to insert standardized codes or forms into appropriate fields in records. Humans are particularly adept at recognizing and correcting errors that are difficult for computer programs to recognize, especially when local knowledge can be applied to the problem at hand. A simple example illustrates this; each element in the following list is intended to represent the word *Street*: Street, street, Str, Str., St, St., Sttreet, Steet. Some of the elements in the preceding list can be substituted easily by both humans and computers; other errors may present a substantial challenge to humans and software systems and thus cause geocoding failures. Such failures should be examined by knowledgeable workers, who are often able to problem solve and apply correction protocols to increase match rates. The process of examination is aided in many cases by modern geocoding software, which provides a match score that can be used to assess the correspondence between an input address and information contained in the GBF (see Figure 2.1).

Status	Score	Side	X	Y	Ref_ID	Pct_along	ARC_Street	Arc_Zone	Address	City	State	Zip
M	100	L	623127.2621	4612937.964	5462	0.0000	200 South Summit Street	52240	200 South Summit Street	Iowa City	IA	52240
M	92	L	623127.2621	4612937.964	5462	0.0000	200 S Summit St.	52240	200 S Sumit St.	Iowa City	IA	52240
M	82	L	623127.2621	4612937.964	5462	0.0000	200 Summit St.	52240	200 Summit St.	Iowa City	IA	52240
M	74	L	623127.2621	4612937.964	5462	0.0000	200 Sumit St.	52240	200 Sumit St.	Iowa City	IA	52240

FIGURE 2.1 Decreasing scores resulting from commonly encountered errors in the input data.

2.2.2.1 Alternative Referents and Spelling Errors

In many instances, locally named references to roads do not correspond to information contained in GBFs because residents in an area typically refer to roads using local terminology (e.g., Main Street vs. Highway 61). These nomenclature variants, however, are often well known and are included in TIGER (Topologically Integrated Geographic Encoding and Referencing) and other street centerline files. In fact, TIGER contains a special record type to record such variant references.[4]

Spelling errors are sometimes more difficult to detect and correct. For example, Main Street and Maim Street are both possible names that would not be flagged by software as an egregious error. A human, however, would recognize the distinction. In other cases, difficulties occur as a consequence of spelling similarities. This well-known problem has been addressed partly through the use of the *soundex* scheme.[5] Soundex is used to access information that is similar in sound (spoken English) but different in spelling and is particularly useful for variation in names. For example, there are numerous variants of Anderson, including Andersson, Andersen, and Anderton. A soundex code is created by specifying the first letter of the name and then following a set of rules that strip out key consonants and letter combinations to permit access through a common code. Anderson reduces to A536, where A is the first letter, and based on soundex rules, M and N are assigned the value of 5, D and T are assigned 3, and R is assigned 6; the remainder of the name is discarded. Figure 2.2 illustrates how soundex can be used to recognize variant spellings of Summit Street. Rules are also specified for treating prefixes, double letters, and short names.

A succinct description of the soundex approach is available at a Web site maintained by the U.S. National Archives and Records Administration (NARA).[5]

2.2.2.2 Abbreviations

Abbreviations are often encountered in the types of administrative data files that are geocoded. Data input personnel will often use abbreviations as a means of saving keystrokes. Generally, this practice is benign because there is an expectation that humans are easily capable of resolving abbreviated entries into their correct, full, form. Moreover, most abbreviations are easily caught by software through the use of synonym lists unless, of course, the abbreviation contains a typographical error. Such cases will typically be flagged for human inspection.

Number	Prefix	Name	Suffix	Zone	Soundex
200	S	Summit	St.	52240	U530
200	S	Sumit	St.	52240	U530
200	S	Summmmit	St.	52240	U530

FIGURE 2.2 Soundex codes for different spelling variants of Summit Street are the same.

2.2.2.3 Prefixes and Suffixes

Prefixes and suffixes that are attached to the core element of a street name can provoke serious problems during address matching. Although prefixes often take a cardinal direction form (East Main), numerous other variants can be observed in practice (e.g., Old vs. New). Suffixes often refer to the type of street referenced, such as Lane or Boulevard. Confusion may occur when the street name and type are the same or similar. For example, Court Street Court is a perfectly plausible street name, but it may be flagged as an error. Careful attention to abbreviation standards must be maintained to reduce these mismatch errors.

2.2.3 GEOGRAPHIC BASE FILES

Information is needed to describe the geographical characteristics of a region in which address matching takes place. This information typically takes one of three forms: administrative jurisdictions (usually polygonal areas), street centerlines, and individual land parcels that may be represented by a polygon or a single coordinate value. Although this information is often accepted as a fait accompli, significant variations in the quality of data can be observed across different data sources. Geographic information quality should be evaluated carefully for completeness and accuracy and to ensure that the data source is fit for its contemplated use. Among the factors to evaluate are

- Compilation method
- Compilation scale and level of generalization
- Date of compilation
- Topological completeness
- Address ranges

The method of compilation used may have significant effects on the accuracy of the product used during geocoding. In some cases, an original survey is conducted, or remote sensing based on digital orthophotography (with geometric distortion removed) may be used. In other cases, data are derived from existing sources or purchased so that they can be modified. It is noteworthy that the number of large geographic data providers is decreasing as a consequence of industrial consolidation.

The scale at which source material is compiled will have significant effects on the level of generalization found in the base file. Detailed maps (low levels of generalization) typically represent linear features with high degrees of fidelity and will capture sinuosity in a line if it is present; generalized representations, on the other hand, will lose sinuosity. Consequently, generalization may play a role when road lengths are considered as part of an address range calculation. For most analytical geographic information system (GIS) applications, a street is represented abstractly as a street centerline. Because residences are not located in the middle of the street, this representation method will cause problems when address-matching results are displayed as maps. In such instances, houses that are directly across a street from each other would be symbolized by overplotting them on the centerline. GIS software typically provides an artificial means for approximating the location of a residence through the use of a parameter that offsets the symbol away from the centerline (e.g., 10 meters). In some urban engineering applications, however, a street must be represented using width (e.g., to map the placement of a water main).

The accuracy of a GBF may be affected by new construction and modifications to the existing road network: If streets do not exist in the GBF, then a match cannot be made. Commercial geographic data providers employ teams that are assigned the task of ensuring that new streets are recorded, and that data already in the system accurately reflect the characteristics of the road network.

Within the context of a GBF, *topology* refers to relative location (adjacent, within). Topological cobounding relations specify whether street segments connect. In addition, GBFs such as the U.S. Census TIGER files attempt to enforce a concept referred to as *parity*: Odd addresses must fall on a single side of a street segment, and even addresses are assigned to the remaining side.

Each street segment in a GBF has a range of addresses associated with it. In some cases, the range accurately represents reality. In other cases, "theoretical" ranges are used. For example, address ranges for blocks may be incremented by 100. Thus, it is a common practice to refer to the "300 block" of a particular street. In many cases, however, this assumption does not hold, and 100 ranges are used inappropriately (e.g., the real range is from 1 to 39, but the range recorded in the base file is 1 to 99). Consequently, the assumed range will introduce proportionality errors in the geocoding process. If an explicit list of valid addresses is available, then this is a generally preferable alternative.

2.3 GEOCODING TYPES

Approaches to geocoding can be placed into the categories described in greater detail in the following sections. Geocoding methods that establish a one-to-one correspondence between a residential address and a coordinate value are called *exact*. Although exact methods may appear to have high levels of accuracy and precision, they are subject to a variety of different types of errors. The other broad class of geocoding methods, *approximation*, uses calculations to estimate a coordinate value that is assigned to an address. This type of geocoding is also subject to error.

2.3.1 APPROXIMATION METHODS

There are two main types of approximation methods for geocoding. The first, *areal*, is used to place each observation into its correct administrative unit. For example, each individual with late-stage cancer can be put into a socioeconomic context by placing the person into a Census Block Group that is associated with 2000 census information. The second approach, *range*, uses interpolation to estimate locations of addresses along block faces that are typically defined between street intersections.

2.3.1.1 Areal Geocoding

When it is important for a project to aggregate individual-level information to predefined administrative units, each observation with an address can be allocated to its correct block face and then allocated to the geographic unit to which it belongs.

This is possible because each block face has associated with it a range of addresses for each side of the street (parity and topology are important in this case). Thus, if a block face forms the border between two census tracts, an address on that street segment would be located in one of the two tracts depending on address parity. This is the general approach developed by the U.S. Bureau of the Census to automate the process of enumerating survey return information. Areal geocoding also can be implemented using parcel information. If a parcel record contains information about the enumeration units in which it lies, then the assignment of an areal geocode is trivial. If such information does not exist, then a parcel coordinate can be used with a point-in-polygon operation. Point-in-polygon algorithms take a coordinate as input and place it into its correct polygon, assuming that the polygon tessellation exhaustively partitions the area of concern.

2.3.1.2 Range Geocoding

Range geocoding has been employed in a wide variety of research settings. The popularity of this approach is due to its flexibility and the low cost of required GBFs (TIGER). Most GIS software performs geocoding using this approach and employs TIGER, TIGER derivatives, or other commercial data products. Range geocoding works by executing the following general sequence of operations:

1. Read a target address and parse it into its constituent elements (e.g., number, prefix, main name, suffix, postal code).
2. Match the target to a street in the GBF using the main name as well as prefixes and suffixes; to improve performance, search is often restricted through the use of postal codes.
3. After the correct street is selected, use the number field in the address to determine the street segment (e.g., between intersections) that contains the address in its range.
4. For that segment, calculate the address range (high–low) stored for the correct side of the street (parity).
5. Establish a proportion by dividing the difference between the minimum address and the target address by the difference between the minimum address and maximum address (the address range) for the correct side of the segment.
6. Determine the difference in coordinates from the endpoints of the street segment; this establishes the geometrical length of the block face (alternatively, use the coordinates that describe the street segment to compute a length by summing interpoint distances).
7. Apply the address proportion calculated in step 5 to the geometry of the segment (step 6) to interpolate a location at a proportional distance between the endpoints.

The use of range geocoding requires the user to make a series of assumptions about the correspondence between what is contained in the GBF and what is present in the real world. The first assumption is that the geometry contained in the file is correct to a degree of accuracy that is commensurate with the application. If the geometry provides a markedly incorrect estimate of length, then the proportion used to interpolate the location of an address will be incorrect. The second assumption is that the address ranges contained in the GBF are correct. As noted, however, departures from this expectation are common. In the neighborhood in which one of the authors resides, for example, house addresses are incremented by 5; in other areas, increments of 10 and 2 are commonly observed. In other cases, addresses have been encoded using ranges that increase by 100 as one moves from block to block, even where there are not 100 addresses present; in fact, it is unusual for 100 physical addresses to be present on a block in many cities. An additional assumption is that the frontage for each address is a constant value. This assumption allows the calculation of location by proportion. However, if the assumption is violated, incorrect locations will be derived. This problem can become significant in modern subdivisions that have modified wedge-shaped parcels that alternate long and short frontages between the back and front of lots. It can also become problematic in areas where large lots are interspersed with smaller lots.

2.3.2 Exact Methods

Exact geocoding methods are becoming more important because of changes in technology and the increasing availability of highly accurate digital cadastral (land ownership) information. The Global Navigation Satellite System (GNSS) approach described in the next section uses satellite location technology to assign a coordinate value to an address. Parcel-based approaches exploit the fact that each parcel has an address that can be represented by a coordinate (e.g., a parcel centroid) and a match (e.g., a *join*) between parcel address and administrative address enables geocoding to occur.

2.3.2.1 GNSS-Based Geocoding

The GNSS is comprised of several interacting systems that are either in place or are in the process of implementation. The Global Positioning System (GPS) has been deployed by the U.S. Department of Defense for more than a decade. GLONASS (a Russian acronym that translates approximately as Global Navigation Satellite System) is a similar system that was implemented by Russia (it originated in the Union of Soviet Socialist Republics [USSR]). In both cases, the basic mission of the systems was to support military operations; civil uses were secondary. More recently, members of the European Union have developed a third civil system called Galileo. All three systems rely on the use of signals sent from satellites placed in precisely monitored orbits. The time distance between when each signal is transmitted from several satellites and when it is received is used to triangulate locations on the surface of the earth (see reference 6). Low-cost receivers can be used by field-workers to record coordinates for residence locations, and geocoding software is used to establish a one-to-one correspondence between the address assigned to each residence and its GNSS-derived coordinate. Although the process of recording such coordinates is labor intensive, the coordinates are typically accurate. Moreover, field-workers can record ancillary information about each address that can be useful in a variety of contexts, such as number of stories, facade type, and the location of outbuildings.

2.3.2.2 Parcel Geocoding

The spatial data infrastructure continues to be developed in most areas of the United States. A key component of this emerging infrastructure is referred to as the *cadastre*. This information describes, at high spatial resolution, the boundaries of land parcels and their attributes. Digital orthophotographs or surveyed boundaries (sometimes with building footprints added) are used to construct this layer of information in a GIS database. Although the polygonal perimeter of each parcel is described, other information is important for geocoding. In particular, a coordinate is normally assigned either to the centroid of the parcel or to the location of the center of a building footprint (e.g., residence) on the parcel. In addition, each parcel has a postal-type address that can be matched against administrative records; when a one-to-one correspondence is found, the coordinate value is transferred.

2.4 AVAILABLE MATERIALS

TIGER line files describe U.S. street centerlines and census geography. This resource, which was developed originally by the U.S. Census Bureau to support their data collection activities, has been used in a variety of ways to support geocoding. Although far from perfectly accurate, TIGER is regularly updated by the Census Bureau and local government agencies. Several commercial firms have developed products that also can be used to support geocoding. These firms also offer value-added products and services, including customized geocoding and improvements to both street centerline geometry and address ranges.

2.4.1 TIGER

When maps are represented in digital form, points, lines, and areas are insufficient for describing relationships that are needed to support geocoding. Consequently, additional information that describes the topological relations among point, line, and area features is encoded. This information helps to form a more complete description of these features. TIGER adopts a specific type of nomenclature to describe map features: zero cells, one cells, and two cells refer to points (zero dimensions), lines (one dimension), and areas (two dimensions), respectively. Zero cells are typically the end nodes of street segments or other linear features described in TIGER. In addition to its geometrical coordinate value, each zero cell may have a list of the one cells that meet at that location. The list therefore would include all the street segments that meet at an intersection. An example of a value-added feature for that intersection would be an additional list that identifies turn restrictions, a so-called turn table.

Each one cell is cobounded by the pair of two cells on each side of it. Each two cell, however, may have several descriptors. For example, a single street segment could serve as a line of separation between census blocks, block groups, and tracts as well as other administrative jurisdictions, such as school districts.

Each side of a one cell also has the key information used to support geocoding: an address range (low address and high address for each side of the street segment). Each address range in TIGER has a single parity. Only odd-numbered addresses are contained within an address range with odd starting and ending numbers (and vice versa). Generally, the left and the right sides of a one cell have opposite parities.

It is important to recall that the actual address ranges for a street segment may depart from those contained in TIGER. These potential address ranges are acceptable for geocoding to areas because any true address will be contained in the specified range for a street segment; errors of omission are reduced as a consequence. However, as described in this chapter, these potential ranges cause geometrical difficulties when interpolated geocoding methods are employed. In such cases, the real addresses are squeezed to the end of the street segment that contains the low address.

2.4.1.1 General Structure

TIGER files are comprised of multiple record types that contain geographic attributes such as address ranges and ZIP codes for complete chains, latitude/longitude coordinates of point features, polygon boundaries, and other information.[4] This multirecord approach is used to increase flexibility of data storage: At each particular location, there may not be a need to have a particular record type, and such information may be omitted to reduce storage requirements. This flexible strategy was adopted in part as a reaction to the limitations associated with a more rigid structure imposed by a TIGER predecessor that was also developed by the U.S. Census Bureau: DIME (dual independent map encoding).

2.4.1.2 TIGER Addresses

An important aspect of TIGER is that it has a goal of containing addresses for each side of every street in the United States. Streets and addresses, however, are constantly changing, and this goal is difficult to achieve as a consequence. One update program was particularly successful prior to the 2000 census: TIGER Improvement Program (TIP). A key element of this program included partnerships with local government agencies. These agencies provided address range "clusters" from the USPS ZIP + 4 file that failed to geocode to the TIGER database. Using local expertise, participants annotated maps derived from TIGER to correct errors and add missing streets, street names, and address ranges. Census staff then incorporated updates into TIGER. As a result of these experiences, the Census Bureau has engaged in partnerships to ensure that their basic information is kept up to date, even during intercensal periods. For Census 2000, the Master Address File (MAF) was introduced. The MAF lists all living quarters nationwide along with their geographic locations. The U.S. Census Bureau created MAF by combining addresses in 1990 TIGER with USPS information. The MAF is maintained through partnerships with USPS, other government agencies, and the private sector. In preparation for the 2010 decennial census, the Census Bureau has initiated a plan for TIGER modernization and enhancement that is focused on increasing the accuracy of locations and change detection.

2.4.1.3 TIGER Limitations

Although TIGER and related derivatives have been used to support a range of successful geocoding activities, a few problems remain. Indeed, its basic structure is inadequate for some applications. One particularly important limitation is that TIGER is planar, but the real world is three dimensional. For example, transportation networks contain nonplanar elements such as overpasses, and the planar structure cannot accommodate such phenomena. Moreover, multistory residences are collapsed to a single point located along a street centerline.

2.4.2 COMMERCIAL GEOGRAPHIC BASE FILES

Several companies provide commercial products that contain geographic information and addresses. There has been a consolidation of these firms. In the following sections, we describe four service providers but make no recommendation about any particular product or company; the companies are mentioned only to illustrate the types of goods and services available. Information in this section was obtained from corporate Web sites.

2.4.2.1 Tele Atlas

Tele Atlas (which was formerly known as ETAK) acquired Geographic Data Technologies (GDT) in 2004. GDT, which had been in business since 1980, was responsible for the development of a geographic database, called Dynamap, and Tele Atlas now provides this product for sale. Dynamap is a continuously updated GBF that is used to support commercial and public sector geocoding activities. Tele Atlas also provides contract geocoding services and provides a commercial online self-service geocoding portal.

2.4.2.2 NAVTEQ

NAVTEQ is a commercial product that is also available through Tele Atlas because it was the main geographic base product provided by ETAK. NAVTEQ is distributed in three levels of content completeness. The database not only contains basic geographic information, but also is used mainly for navigational purposes and contains information about turn restrictions and limited access highways. The NAVTEQ database is also continuously updated and checked for correctness.

2.4.2.3 Google

Google has entered the geocoding arena and provides an applications programming interface (API) that requests a geocoding result when an address is submitted to the Google service. Google claims that it is not necessary to split addresses into constituent parts; instead, a single string can be submitted. Moreover, it translates abbreviations into full strings. In addition to a mapped result, it is also possible to obtain a formatted and parsed version of the input address along with a latitude and longitude coordinate (elevation is always set to zero). At the present time, Google is imposing a geocoding limit of 50,000 addresses each day. It is important to note that Google is a service provider and does not create GBF content; for that, Google relies on both NAVTEQ and Tele Atlas.

2.4.2.4 Yahoo!

Yahoo! also provides an API that can be used either to obtain geographic coordinates for a given address string or to map an address directly using an AJAX (Asynchronous JavaScript and XML [extensible markup language])/Flash interface. In addition to returning latitude and longitude information, the API also returns the address in a standardized format along with the precision of the resulting geocode (address, street, ZIP, city, state or country). The results are returned as an XML document from which relevant information can be parsed. As of August 2006, the service is limited to 5000 queries per IP (Internet protocol) address per day. Like Google, Yahoo! also relies on external providers for its GBF content.

2.5   TOWARD A GEOCODING ERROR BUDGET

Although reliable and robust geocoding software has been refined over a period of several decades, geocoding is rarely a fully automated process. Errors and failures are difficult to detect using automated approaches, but they are often easily treated by personnel, especially those who have received some training in geocoding. Such training enables them to understand why different types of errors occur and to select appropriate remediation strategies. Researchers who intend to geocode data, or use the results of geocoding, should know about likely problems and the ways that users can treat these problems, including effects on the quality and reliability of results.

We begin by assuming that there is an input digital file (the source) that contains thematic information with no locational identifiers other than a thoroughfare address. This information is then transformed through the addition of one or more geocodes that allow the information to be mapped or analyzed geographically. Maps may be created through the addition of a coordinate or an areal geocode, which supports aggregation to defined polygonal units such as census tracts or to areas that are artifacts of analytical procedures. Each transformation of source information will typically introduce errors of omission and commission. In general, an address may not geocode because of inaccuracies or inconsistencies in the digital street map or in the source file of addresses to be matched. The proportion of addresses correctly matched, often referred to as the *hit rate*, will increase if efforts are made to increase the quality of the GBF, the source address file, or both.

2.5.1   GEOGRAPHIC BASE FILE ERRORS

The form of the GBF will vary by type of geocoding method employed. For the typical interpolated form of geocoding, the base file consists of a topologically structured road centerline file with address ranges and geographic area codes (e.g., census units, congressional district) that are assigned to each side of a street segment. In this form, geometrical errors can occur when the street is improperly represented by coordinates; in TIGER, this geometrical description is specified by so-called shape

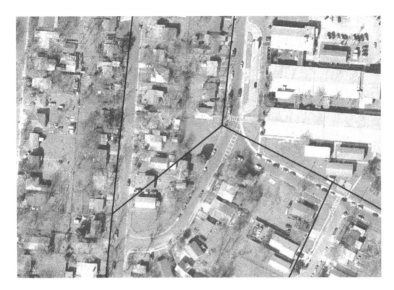

FIGURE 2.3 A generalized road segment in TIGER data coarsely approximates the sinuosity present in the actual road network.

points that in many cases provide only a general characterization of geometrical form. Although a limited number of shape points is not problematic where places have a rectilinear network (only two points are needed to represent a straight line), the absence of geometrical fidelity can introduce errors if the road segment has considerable sinuosity (Figure 2.3). In such cases, the estimated geocode will be a coarse approximation, and any other distance calculations that use the network coordinates will be inaccurate. This type of error can be corrected through the use of ungeneralized maps (often derived from orthophotographs) or through the use of GPS-based observations, often obtained by driving along streets and subsequent application of geometrical smoothing algorithms to reduce GPS-derived variability in location.

Topological errors also cause serious problems during geocoding and other uses of GBFs. The most glaring topological error occurs when a road segment is missing. This can occur as a consequence of data input errors or may result from data that are not maintained or updated to reflect new construction. In either case, an address that is correct in the source database cannot be assigned to its correct location along a street because either the street or street segment does not exist in the GBF. In other cases, connections are identified where none exist. Such errors are relatively uncommon and typically do not cause enormous problems during geocoding. However, such errors can have a substantial effect on other uses of the GBF, especially routing and distance calculations. In general, these error types can be identified by field checking or by digitizing from updated sources when new construction occurs. As mentioned, the TIGER line data set and all commercial products are frequently updated. Figure 2.4 highlights those street segments that were added to the TIGER data set for the Iowa City/Coralville area in Iowa over the 10-year period between 1990 and 2000.

In some cases, as shown in Figure 2.5, line segments that represent road networks may be incorrectly digitized. Such errors may increase the geocoding hit

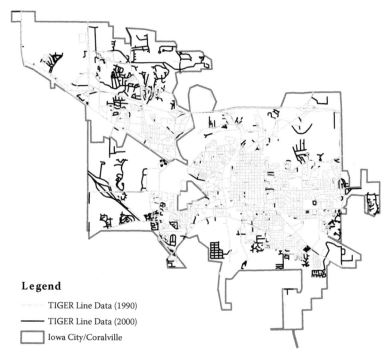

FIGURE 2.4 The dark lines indicate all those street segments that were added to the TIGER data set for the Iowa City/Coralville area over a 10-year period from 1990 to 2000.

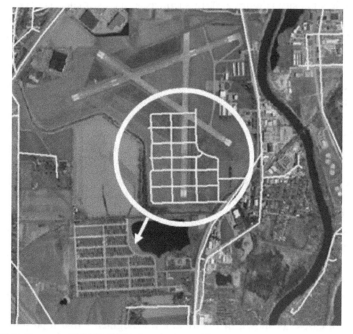

FIGURE 2.5 Errors in TIGER/2000 data for Iowa City, Iowa.

rate and hence the users' confidence in the GBF. However, they can have serious consequences on the accuracy of the geocodes obtained. Checking for such errors using freely available orthoimagery is a fairly straightforward but labor-intensive task. Consequently, it is often neglected by users, who make assumptions about the geometrical quality of the GBFs.

As we discussed, road networks in a GBF are usually represented as street centerlines. When addresses are geocoded using such data, it is common map-making practice to offset the geocodes from the street centerline by some constant value. This may be an acceptable practice in urban areas, where residences and other buildings are usually constrained by the availability of space. However, in rural areas, farms and other buildings may be constructed at varying distances away from the street centerlines. To further complicate this problem, street centerlines in the TIGER data often do not fall exactly in the center of the actual road. Figure 2.6A shows

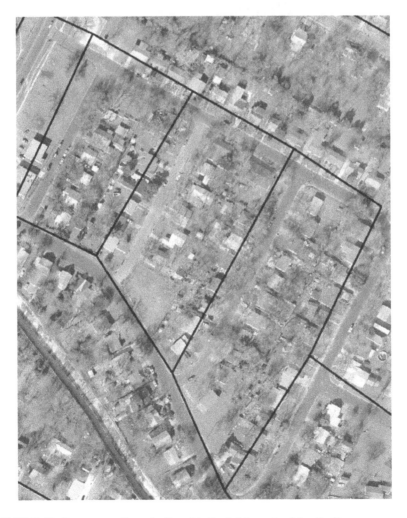

FIGURE 2.6A Street centerline misaligned to the left in parts of Austin, Texas.

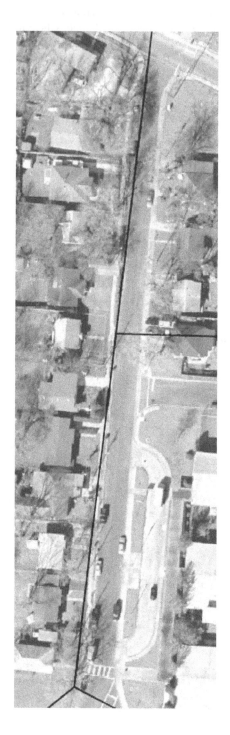

FIGURE 2.6B Street centerline shifts disproportionately as it moves from the top of this street segment to the bottom.

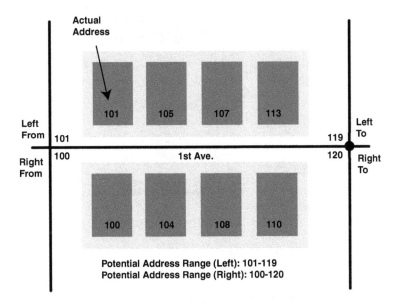

Potential Address Range (Left): 101-119
Potential Address Range (Right): 100-120

FIGURE 2.7 Potential address range encoding. (Redrawn from TIGER/Line® Technical Documentation, 2nd ed., 2004; prepared by the U.S. Census Bureau, 2005.)

street centerlines in Austin, Texas, that are misaligned toward the left side of the actual road segments. Figure 2.6B is an example of a street centerline that shifts to the left as it goes from the top to the bottom of the street segment. In such situations, constant offset distances may bias the geocodes in one direction or the other.

The specific location of a geocode along a street segment is determined by interpolating the address number along the line that represents that particular street given a potential address range defined *a priori* (Figure 2.7). This process often works well in urban and suburban areas, where a regular ordering of structures along a particular street segment can be observed. However, as in the preceding case, in rural areas this method of establishing a geocoded location often fails to provide good geographical accuracy.

In the example shown in Figure 2.8, we employ TIGER/2000 data and ArcGIS software to geocode an address numbered 28734. The potential address range for the street on which this residence is located is encoded as 28738 to 28400. The geocoding mechanism in the GIS software interpolates this address number along the street line segment and places a point at one end of the line. When this location is compared to the actual location of the residence determined using high-resolution orthoimagery for the area, we find that the geocode for the given address was placed approximately 450 meters away from the actual location of the residence (Figure 2.8). The problem, of course, is not the software or the geocoding methods, but the incorrect specification of the potential address range for that particular street segment. Although proper encoding of address ranges will eliminate such errors, updating TIGER data with specific information for each street is often labor intensive, involving manually correcting geocodes using high-resolution orthoimagery or GPS measurements.

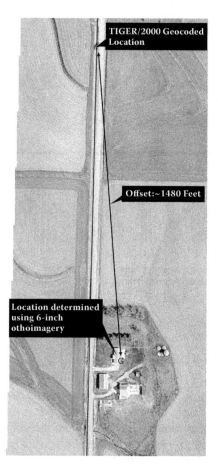

FIGURE 2.8 Geocoding errors caused by incorrect address range encoding in the TIGER data.

In addition to such range problems, other attribute and data errors in GBFs are significant contributors to the overall geocoding error budget. We demonstrate the impacts of these types of geocoding errors using the TIGER/2000 data for Carroll County, Iowa, which is a rural county with a population of approximately 22,000. The largest city has a population of approximately 10,000 and covers 5.5 square miles. All towns and cities in Carroll County have a single, unique ZIP code. We queried the TIGER data for all street segments where the street name was 2nd street and the ZIP code was 51455 (Manning, IA). Our query, however, returned results from the opposite sides of the county (Figure 2.9).

On examining the attribute data in more detail, we discovered that the TIGER line data for Carroll County had incorrect ZIP codes defined for some of its streets. On examining these data further, we found that roughly 10% of the street segments in this data set had ZIP codes defined as 66441, which is the ZIP code for Junction City, Kansas (Figure 2.10). ZIP code errors are important because these codes are often used by geocoding software to restrict a search to a local area.

The darker lines represent the results of the query:
Street Name = '2nd Street' and Zip (Left) = '51455'

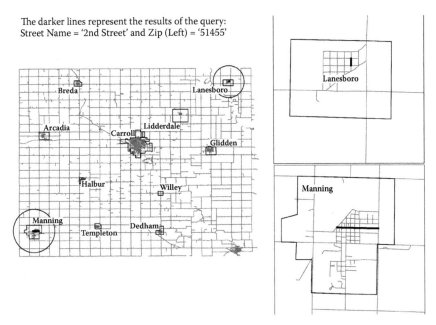

FIGURE 2.9 Map showing the location of ZIP code errors.

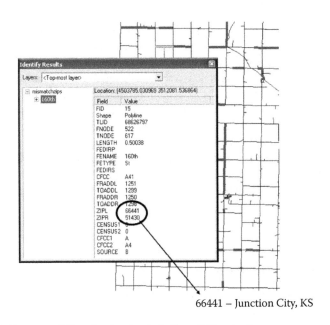

66441 – Junction City, KS

FIGURE 2.10 Incorrect ZIP codes for streets in Carroll County, Iowa.

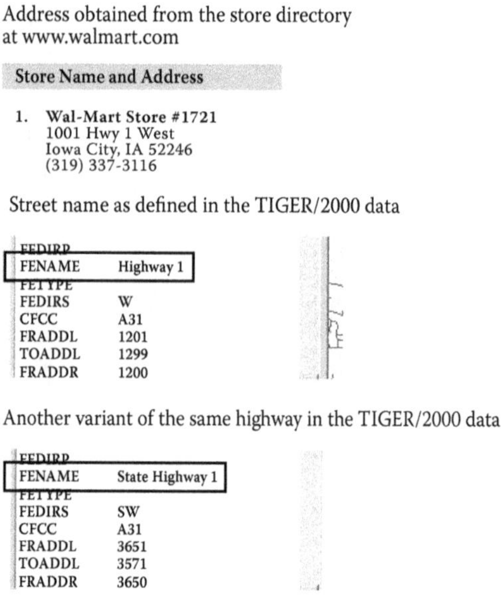

Address obtained from the store directory
at www.walmart.com

Store Name and Address

1. **Wal-Mart Store #1721**
    1001 Hwy 1 West
    Iowa City, IA 52246
    (319) 337-3116

Street name as defined in the TIGER/2000 data

FEDIRP	
FENAME	Highway 1
FETYPE	
FEDIRS	W
CFCC	A31
FRADDL	1201
TOADDL	1299
FRADDR	1200

Another variant of the same highway in the TIGER/2000 data

FEDIRP	
FENAME	State Highway 1
FETYPE	
FEDIRS	SW
CFCC	A31
FRADDL	3651
TOADDL	3571
FRADDR	3650

FIGURE 2.11 Examples of street name variations.

2.5.2 ADDRESS ERRORS

Apart from problems in the GBFs, data entry errors and the naming conventions used in the input data sets can also be important contributors to geocoding error. Data entry errors include incorrect spellings and unwanted spaces. Some errors of this type can be easily fixed using spell-checkers now commonly available in database and spreadsheet packages. The problems caused by local naming conventions, however, are much harder to resolve. We attempted to geocode the address of a local Wal-Mart store in Iowa City, Iowa, using TIGER/2000 data and ArcGIS. The address of this store's location was obtained from the official Wal-Mart Web site. As shown in Figure 2.11, the official naming convention for Highway 1 West in the TIGER data set is different from that used on the Wal-Mart Web site. The result, of course, was a failed geocode. Addresses with such disparities are routinely stored in administrative data sets for the purposes of recording address information. Geocoding such addresses using GBFs that typically adhere to more formal naming conventions can have a serious impact on the geocoding hit rate. In most cases, such errors need to be manually examined and fixed.

2.5.2.1 Duplicate Addresses

Many administrative data sets not only contain erroneous data but also contain many duplicate addresses. When these duplicate addresses can be discarded, they can be easily removed using commonly available spreadsheet and database packages. However, in other situations these duplicate addresses may be important and cannot be discarded. For example, consider a health data set in which each record corresponds to a unique health event from the same residential address. If errors in such data sets need to be corrected manually, then the process of dealing with many duplicate addresses that have the same error is extremely inefficient. One solution to this problem is to generate a unique ID for each address in the data set based on the address string itself. These IDs can then be used not only to eliminate duplicate addresses from the data set but also to link information back to the original data set when needed. These IDs also provide an efficient way to link multiple data sets that share common records. A common way of creating such IDs uses a method called *hash functions*. A hash function maps strings of an arbitrary length (such as a postal address) to small binary strings of a fixed length, known as *hash values*. There are many different algorithms that can be employed to generate such hash values. The SHA1 algorithm is commonly used.[7] Although it is unlikely, it has been shown that in certain special cases the SHA1 algorithm is not "strongly collision free." This means that with large computation resources, it is possible to find two different input strings (such as addresses) that can produce the same hash value or ID. However, newer variants of the SHA1 algorithm that use a longer word size, which is the number of bytes that can be processed by a computer at one time, are known to be strongly collision free. One such variant is the SHA-256/224. In the example in Figure 2.12, we use the SHA1 algorithm to generate the hash IDs for a given set of addresses.

2.5.2.2 Incorrectly Formatted Addresses

In rare cases, the source file may contain addresses that are incorrectly formatted. For example, a file could be produced by a database that is sorted on the basis of ZIP code and that would be the first field written. In other cases, city names might appear first. When such files are encountered, the format must first be determined, and then the file is transformed into the expected sequence, typically using a DBMS or spreadsheet software.

2.5.2.3 Postal Addresses

Many residents in the United States elect to have mail delivered to central facilities such as post offices or drop boxes provided by private companies. Consequently, when records contain fields for billing or other postal delivery functions, the residential address is not provided. In such cases, the records cannot be geocoded to yield home locations. This introduces problems because large proportions of geocoded results are, strictly speaking, placed at the location of the mail facility, thus causing error in any analysis that would be conducted with the geocoded results.

Procedures can be established to distribute these erroneous assignments.

1. Ancillary information can be used to obtain street addresses. Telephone directories and other sources can be used to determine street addresses for some of the individuals who use a post office box. This approach, however, also has its own set of limitations. Many people do not publish their telephone listing. Moreover, a person trying to establish a link between the sources will be forced to assume a correspondence between the names of people in the sources consulted. Names, however, are inadequate as unique identifiers. This is also a very labor-intensive process.
2. Individuals who use post office boxes can be randomly assigned to an address list or to street segments. In the absence of other information, this

Original Data

ADDRESS	HASHID
10463 QUARTZ AVE	//+muNFZ3yGe/koqH5f5FBpA123ZsPdwh+SCVJdixiu4njRz9pEDtdQsk/VuMsVIrq0Pxo4RxlFhF6/RLpZaK2w==
31593 VELVET AVE	//2aa0+FINJD+RI1VJ4mWrXLvcdNQwZDnHF+LJ3uwXqsc1 xfruzF7jh4crGL3NS9CVkGlngR2LCDawmXakiyQ==
31593 VELVET AVE	//2aa0+FINJD+RI1VJ4mWrXLvcdNQwZDnHF+LJ3uwXqsc1 xfruzF7jh4crGL3NS9CVkGlngR2LCDawmXakiyQ==
31593 VELVET AVE	//2aa0+FINJD+RI1VJ4mWrXLvcdNQwZDnHF+LJ3uwXqsc1 xfruzF7jh4crGL3NS9CVkGlngR2LCDawmXakiyQ==
31593 VELVET AVE	//2aa0+FINJD+RI1VJ4mWrXLvcdNQwZDnHF+LJ3uwXqsc1 xfruzF7jh4crGL3NS9CVkGlngR2LCDawmXakiyQ==
31593 VELVET AVE	//2aa0+FINJD+RI1VJ4mWrXLvcdNQwZDnHF+LJ3uwXqsc1 xfruzF7jh4crGL3NS9CVkGlngR2LCDawmXakiyQ==

Non-duplicate data for geocoding purposes

ADDRESS	HASHID
10463 QUARTZ AVE	//+muNFZ3yGe/koqH5f5FBpA123ZsPdwh+SCVJdixiu4njRz9pEDtdQskVuMsVIrq0Pxo4RxlFhF6/RLpZzK2w==
31593 VELVET AVE	//2aa0+FINJD+RI1VJ4mWrXLvcdNQwZDnHF+LJ3uwXqsc1 xfruzF7jh4crGL3NS9CVkGlngR2LCDawmXakiyQ==
773 7TH AVE	//YVVvUJpy7wBAoVEhCAjxEJr6Hw1qstQr+UoVM4Lbb36sajREt/qhefIFurky2qtGGM9XDoQltZgm2/+nd08lg==
1511 BIRCH ST	/+abolok16pzn12ff6azKdAj2GyNvdffI1w86el/GfO26aXEHRLSNmacZtrmvVCihp86Co6BcSmoYJjOGus+Q==
16268 HWY 141	/08e93dhdssMVAjJlmWe6K5Z6kabEMb1815Xjt1bKErzCjifDvg1t1mL3NQ3y5m0MQhpjgV4rNrn/0zahaRk8w==
604 OAK	/0gOra0kUygygebP7lholKlwingm2FAm/MpAL4XGKMmG1mnq8L8iviat13U4ySAN5b4AKKmO8orBio8OmCCalS6A==

FIGURE 2.12 Use of hash IDs to eliminate duplicate records for geocoding purposes.

may produce acceptable results if aggregation is used to create variables for further analysis. The assumption of uniformity, however, is tenuous.

3. Assignment may be made to a weighted location. In this case, probabilities of assignment are derived from variables that describe the characteristics of an area. For example, population density could be used to influence the location of assignment. An alternative would be to create a model of post office box usage based on socioeconomic characteristics and to use results of the model to influence assignments.

None of these procedures is an attractive alternative. The use of post office boxes is likely to remain a vexing problem for those attempting to use geocoding to establish locational information for individuals.

2.6 CONCLUSION

Geocoding can be a valuable tool if it is used properly to support spatial analysis of health information. Geocoding software is widely available, and GBFs are also available from a variety of sources. Nevertheless, geocoding processes can be error prone, and the results of subsequent analyses will be adversely affected by geocoding errors. In this chapter, we have described commonly employed geocoding methods and data materials. Given the importance of data quality on results, we have placed a particular emphasis on documenting the types of errors that are likely to be encountered in any geocoding project. Such knowledge can be used to improve procedures that are implemented to detect and eliminate errors, which will lead in turn to higher quality analytical results.

REFERENCES

1. Dueker, K. J. 1974. Urban Geocoding. *Annals of the Association of American Geographers* 64:318–325.
2. Address Standards Working Group. 2005. *Street Address Data Standard* (Working Draft 2.0). Federal Geographic Data Committee: 134. http://www.fgdc.gov/standards/projects/FGDC-standards-projects/street-address/05-11.2ndDraft.CompleteDoc.pdf
3. U.S. Postal Service. 2006. Postal Addressing Standards Publication 28. http://pe.usps.gov/cpim/ftp/pubs/pub28/pub28.pdf
4. Broome, F. R., and D. B. Meixler. 1990. The TIGER data base structure. *Cartography and Geographic Information Systems* 17:39–48.
5. U.S. National Archives and Records Administration. 2007. The soundex indexing system. http://www.archives.gov/genealogy/census/soundex.html
6. Rizos, C. 2002. Introducing the global positioning system. In J.D. Bossler, J.R. Jensen, and R.B. McMaster (Eds). *Manual of Geospatial Science and Technology*. New York: Taylor & Francis, pp. 77–94.
7. Federal Information Processing Standards. 2002. *Secure Hash Standard (SHS)* (FIPS Publication 180-2). U.S. DoC/NIST.

3 Using ZIP® Codes as Geocodes in Cancer Research

Kirsten M. M. Beyer, Alan F. Schultz,
and Gerard Rushton

CONTENTS

3.1   INTRODUCTION

Although the ZIP code has many advantages as a geographic unit to use when mapping health data, such as its widespread accessibility as a geocode in health databases and its small spatial size, it also has a number of limitations, such as the fact that true boundaries of ZIP codes are not known and change through time. It is well known that the choice of geographic unit can affect the interpretation of maps and the results of spatial analyses, a phenomenon known as the *modifiable areal unit problem* (MAUP).[1] As such, it is important to consider the advantages and disadvantages of the ZIP code, as well as other geographical units, before deciding on a unit that will yield the most accurate maps and analysis of cancer data. In this chapter, we examine the advantages and disadvantages of the ZIP code, explore examples of research that have used the ZIP code, and address key questions about ZIP code use.

3.2 ADVANTAGES AND DISADVANTAGES OF THE ZIP CODE IN CANCER MAPPING

The ZIP code is fundamentally a tool of the U.S. Postal Service (USPS) and was developed for purposes of facilitating the delivery of mail. According to the U.S. Census Bureau, a ZIP (Zone Improvement Plan) code is "the numerical code assigned by the USPS to designate a local area or entity for the delivery of mail."[2] Difficulties in using this unit for mapping stem from the fact that the ZIP code was developed for the specific purpose of delivering mail, and thus its development did not take into consideration problems that may arise in utilizing the ZIP code in data collection, presentation, or analysis.

A fundamental problem in using the ZIP code for mapping is the fact that true spatial boundaries of ZIP codes are not generally known. In fact, if they were known, some geographic areas represented by a single ZIP code would not be contiguous areas. This is because the geographic areas represented by ZIP codes are based on delivery routes, not land areas. According to the U.S. Census Bureau, ZIP codes "are networks of streets served by mail carriers or just individual post offices."[3] The USPS has never delineated the geographic boundaries of ZIP codes, making it less useful for those for whom knowing the exact area it serves is important. Commercial firms have delineated ZIP code boundaries through interpolation,[3-5] although the accuracy of these boundaries regarding mail delivery by ZIP code is not guaranteed,[3] and they have been criticized for representational error.[6]

Census data were tabulated for five-digit ZIP codes for the 1970, 1980, and 1990 U.S. censuses. For the year 2000 census, the U.S. Census Bureau created a new entity called the ZIP Code Tabulation Area (ZCTA™) and made boundary files for these areas available. In addition, the U.S. Census Bureau discontinued tabulating population data by ZIP code, tabulating instead by ZCTA. The problem with using the ZCTA as a geographic unit for the presentation of health data collected by ZIP code is that the ZCTA boundaries do not coincide with the true boundaries of the ZIP code, and thus health events collected by ZIP code could potentially be misplaced. This could occur because of the way ZCTAs are created. According to the U.S. Census Bureau, ZCTAs are "generalized area representations" of ZIP code areas and are created by aggregating all census blocks for which the majority five-digit ZIP code is the same.[7] Thus, locations that have a ZIP code that is in the minority in a census block will be assigned a ZCTA code that does not correspond with their ZIP code. For those areas where it is difficult to determine the prevailing five-digit ZIP code, the higher-level three-digit ZIP code is used for the ZCTA code.[7]

Because the true boundaries of ZIP codes are not known, it is problematic to assume, for example, that cancer cases and population data for the same individual are assigned to the same area. Whereas a cancer registry collects the ZIP code for an individual, the U.S. Census Bureau collects population data by ZCTAs. This results in spatial misalignment of numerator (cancer cases) and denominator (population data). For example, if an individual's ZIP code is in the minority, the individual will be counted as population in a ZCTA that does not correspond to that individual's ZIP code. Likewise, if the individual has a minority ZIP code and suffers from late-stage colorectal cancer, a late-stage colorectal cancer case will be assigned to one ZCTA (via ZIP code information collected by a cancer registry), and the person's presence will be assigned as population data to another ZCTA. This introduces error into the determination of cancer rates for ZIP code areas.

Another problem that researchers encounter when using the ZIP code to map cancer data is that ZIP codes themselves are not stable through time. ZIP codes are discontinued and introduced to facilitate the delivery of mail,[1] and populations of ZIP codes can change frequently. ZIP code boundaries are more prone to change in parts of the United States experiencing rapid population growth[4] as mail delivery must adjust to changes in population distribution and density. However, it should be noted that other potential choices of areal unit, such as the census tract, also experience boundary changes,[8] although not as frequently as the ZIP code because they are not updated as frequently. As Krieger et al. noted, changes in census tract and block group boundaries over time can be addressed by merging and disaggregating these units to create comparable units, and these methods cannot be employed with ZIP codes.[9]

Often, in mapping cancer data collected over the span of a number of years, one will encounter a cancer case linked to a ZIP code that is no longer in service. It is necessary then to address this problem. Although some have discussed eliminating these records from the data set,[10,11] one approach that preserves health records linked to discontinued ZIP codes in the data set is the reassignment of health records to current ZIP codes. Even though there is the potential for error in performing reassignment, the potential loss of cases may be a more serious problem.

In addition, ZIP code populations can change relatively quickly, making base populations somewhat unstable and complicating the calculation of rates. However, as Carretta and Mick argued, "[ZIP codes] reflect population change more quickly than census tracts [which] appear more stable only because they are updated less frequently."[8] They noted that any pairing of temporally mismatched data (e.g., health events from one year and population data from another) will result in problems regardless of which geographic unit is used, and that updated ZIP code population information is available from commercial firms.[8]

A consideration for any researcher attempting to use the ZIP code to map phenomena that cross state borders is that ZIP codes are not the same size from state to state. There can be large differences in base populations, which results in differences in resolution and statistical stability of maps that utilize approximate ZIP code area borders, thus affecting interpretation of the resultant maps. For example, the number of ZCTAs in New York State is less than twice the number in Iowa (1677 compared to 972), yet New York's 2000 population was roughly 6.5 times bigger than Iowa's (18,976,457 compared to 2,926,324).[12–15]

Finally, as the ZIP code was defined for purposes of mail delivery, it does not deliberately represent a community of interest as census tracts often do. Census tracts are "designed to be relatively homogeneous with respect to population characteristics, economic status, and living conditions (p. 1100)."[10] Krieger et al. used data from Massachusetts and Rhode Island to investigate the merits of area-based measures (census tract, ZIP code, and census block group) in identifying socioeconomic gradients in health outcomes and found that although block group and tract measures performed comparably, ZIP code measures for several outcomes "detected no gradients or gradients contrary to those observed with tract and block group measures (p. 471)."[11] This conclusion was drawn after the elimination of a large number of records because they were geocoded with ZIP codes that no longer existed. On the other hand, Thomas et al. included both ZIP code and census tract income measures in exploratory modeling of a number of causes of mortality across 14 states and found that although census tract-based income was a slightly stronger mortality predictor than ZIP code-based income, both were significant, independent, and "approximately equal" predictors of mortality.[16] The relative merits of demographic measures based on census tract, block group, and ZIP code geography is an ongoing debate, and researchers should look to the literature to provide guidance in determining when the use of ZIP code level data is appropriate.

Despite these limitations, the ZIP code does offer compelling reasons for its use in mapping health data. The main advantages of the ZIP code are its size and availability. ZIP codes represent small geographic areas, which allow for high-quality maps offering more local detail than those relying on the county or other large geographical units. Although Krieger et al. noted that the average population size of ZIP codes in the United States is 30,000, as compared to averages of 4000 for census tracts and 1000 for census block groups,[10] population sizes of ZIP codes vary widely across the country. In 2000 in Illinois, 27.5% of ZIP code areas had fewer than 1000 people, and 56.5% had fewer than 3000 according to Wang.[17] In 2000, Iowa's population was 2,926,324, and there were 949 land-based ZCTAs, making an average population of 3080 per five-digit ZIP code.[12]

The geographic detail attainable with the use of ZIP codes enables a more thorough understanding of the health phenomenon of interest, as well as more effective targeting of intervention geographically, than that offered by larger units such as the county. As the areal unit employed affects the results of geographical study, the choice of an areal unit appropriate for the scale of the phenomenon investigated is critical to the validity of the results.[1] There is a growing body of literature that focuses on the role of community-level factors in affecting health outcomes, making the use of small geographic units ever more important.[18,19]

In addition, the ZIP code is usually known and reported and is thus included in many databases of interest.[1] As such, it may be more widely available for a study population than other geocodes.[16] When an individual accesses health care (e.g., to report an illness, undergo treatment, etc.), the individual is usually capable of reporting his or her address, ZIP code, and county. The county often represents an area too large to use in determining true, local patterns of disease, and the address requires additional geocoding to obtain census block, census tract, or latitude and longitude information. This process represents an additional expense to either the data provider or the researcher.[16]

In addition, the ZIP code may be a more complete geocode than others, such as the census tract or block group, in cancer registry data. We explore the Iowa cancer database as an example. According to Iowa Cancer Registry staff, the ZIP code data are "almost 100% complete and accurate." The ZIP codes attached to registry data in Iowa are edited using a lookup table maintained on the ATLAS database, which is a database developed by the registry in 1988 to standardize the spelling of Iowa towns and provide information for each Iowa city, such as the five-digit ZIP code and the county code. The only exceptions to this are in large cities with more than one ZIP code, because these are not edited, and the incidental changes in rural areas if mail delivery is switched to a different, nearby town. The registry does not evaluate their data and retroactively update ZIP codes. For registry data, the census tract is obtained through geocoding, and a "census tract certainty" code is assigned to each case to indicate how likely it is that the case has been geocoded to the correct census tract. Cases from 1996 to 2004 are geocoded to year 2000 census tracts. Of the total data records, 90.79% (135,302 records) include the complete and valid address of the affected individual and are given an accuracy code of 1. The remaining records are geocoded based on less-complete address information (such as ZIP + 4, ZIP + 2, ZIP only, and post office box) and are coded in decreasing likelihood of obtaining the correct census tract code.[20]

Finally, in a time when the potentially conflicting goals of protecting personal privacy regarding health data and attaining fine geographic detail in mapping and analysis are both prominent, the ZIP code offers a geographic unit that moves toward achieving both. It is common in the literature that a researcher will obtain data at the ZIP code or other level of aggregation instead of the individual level because the data holder is more willing to release the data in aggregated form for privacy reasons. Thus, some argue that the ZIP code does allow both the protection of personal privacy in data use and the achievement of highly detailed maps.[4]

However, it must be noted that according to the definitions put forth in the privacy rule issued pursuant to the Health Insurance Portability and Accountability Act (HIPAA) of 1996, the ZIP code does not go far enough in masking individuals' locations. The HIPAA Privacy Rule sets forth certain requirements for deidentification of what it refers to as protected health information. These requirements include removal of all geographic identifiers smaller than the state[21] except for the first three digits of a ZIP code if

(1) The geographic unit formed by combining all zip codes with the same three initial digits contains more than 20,000 people; and (2) The initial three digits of a zip code for all such geographic units containing 20,000 or fewer people is changed to 000.[22]

Thus, for most small-area mapping, another approach to data sharing must be used, which requires that a qualified person determine that the risk of the geographic information used to identify an individual is small.[23] It is our experience, and that of other researchers,[5,24] that keepers of health data are much more willing to release records that are geocoded to the ZIP code than those geocoded to individual residences. In addition, small ZIP codes can be combined, or smoothing techniques can be used to create maps with stable local detail that effectively preserve personal privacy.[4,17]

Although the ZIP code suffers from serious limitations, it is widely available in health databases with high completeness and accuracy and offers a partial compromise between privacy protection and geographic detail. It is thus a widely used geocode in health research. This is the subject of our next section.

3.3 ZIP CODES IN HEALTH RESEARCH

Use of the ZIP code in health research is widespread. In this section, we discuss examples from health studies that have taken advantage of the ZIP code for use in mapping and analysis and show how different types of studies have made considerable progress using ZIP codes.

The ZIP code has been used in a number of studies focusing on cancer. Johnson (2004) described the use of the ZIP code as a unit of analysis for mapping prostate cancer patterns in New York State, noting that the ZIP code is the chosen unit of analysis for a number of reasons, including that it offers the opportunity to find balance between protecting confidentiality and creating fine-resolution maps.[4] Johnson described how spatial smoothing of population-based measures of disease can be used to overcome one of the limitations of ZIP codes as a unit of analysis — that of the differing population sizes of ZIP codes within a study area.[4] In justifying his choice of the ZIP code, Johnson described a personal communication with the New York State Cancer Registry, by which he was informed that New York had relatively stable ZIP code service areas over the time period of his study (1990–99), with the closure of only 50 small post offices and the addition of 3 new post offices. He noted: "ZIP codes were combined in instances where service delivery area changed between 1990 and 1999 or for confidentiality reasons where necessary."[4]

Again in New York, Jacquez and Greiling used ZIP codes in their two-part analysis of cancer clusters in Long Island and the potential links between risk from exposure to airborne carcinogens and cancer. The New York State Department of Health provided cancer data for the study aggregated by ZIP code to protect privacy. Jacquez and Greiling noted that populations of the ZIP codes ranged widely, from 445 to 105,723 people, and that the populations within ZIP code areas were not uniform with respect to ethnicity or age.[5] For this study, the authors utilized ZIP code area boundary files purchased from a commercial firm.[5] The authors noted that for estimation of individual exposure to airborne carcinogens, both ZIP codes and census tracts provided too coarse a resolution, and that other units may be more suited for estimation of environmental exposure, such as watersheds or "windsheds" in the case of airborne substances.[25] In related work, Goovaerts and Jacquez investigated the validity of the assumption of complete spatial randomness in statistical analyses that seek spatial patterns, using the case of lung cancer by ZIP code in Long Island, New York.[26]

In their study of pancreatic cancer mortality and pesticide exposure in California, Clary and Ritz used mortality data aggregated to the ZIP code (residences on death certificates were only provided at the ZIP code level) along with pesticide exposure data, which was provided at the 1-square-mile (section) level.[27] They then broke down the ZIP code areas by quartiles based on pesticide exposure and calculated mortality risk. They noted that, because ZIP code boundaries change, they could potentially have introduced error into their calculations simply by aggregating exposure data without taking historical boundaries into account. In addition, ZIP codes of residences close to agricultural fields where pesticide use is more concentrated, but not containing them, were not counted as having an increased risk of exposure, which could affect results, although they noted that this would most likely bias the overall estimates toward the null.[27]

White and Aldrich used the ZIP code in an analysis of pediatric cancer risk near hazardous waste sites. They noted that, in determining the areas in which national priorities list (NPL) hazardous waste sites are located, there were some discrepancies among three sources of ZIP code data (the Agency for Toxic Substances and Disease Registry (ATSDR) Internet site, the North Carolina Department of Solid Waste files, and the North Carolina Central Cancer Registry cancer cluster report files), which made locating 25% of the NPL sites complicated.[28] This problem was overcome using United States Geological Survey (USGS) topographic maps to plot site locations and the overlaying of this map with ZIP code area boundaries. In justifying their use of ZIP codes, they noted: "Any health effect produced hypothetically by the NPL site would be lost in the spatial volume of the county, unless the risk level was immense (p. 394)," and that the main benefit of an ecological study such as theirs is to accomplish the analysis with ease and to point researchers in the direction of a more advanced study.[28]

Researchers with the National Cancer Data Base (NCDB), which is a project of the American College of Surgeons Commission on Cancer and the American Cancer Society, utilized ZIP codes to investigate the relationship between breast cancer and the average family income of the ZIP code of residence. This study was undertaken using data from 1995 and 1996, when the U.S. Census Bureau still tabulated economic information by ZIP code. The authors noted that using the average family income of a case's ZIP code of residence is problematic because income levels within ZIP codes can vary.[29]

Nash et al. used the ZIP code to evaluate the effectiveness of an intervention to increase colorectal cancer screening in New York City. They found that individuals screened at the facility of interest — Lincoln Hospital — resided in 48 surrounding ZIP codes in four New York City boroughs. They compared observed and desired numbers of screenings performed, obtaining the desired numbers of screenings performed by age-adjusting estimates based on demographic characteristics of each ZIP code.[30]

Wang used the ZIP code to investigate the spatial distribution of cancer in Illinois. He used the ZIP code because he sought a finer resolution than that offered by the county for purposes of cluster detection; however, as he noted that mapping rare diseases such as cancer using small areas such as ZIP codes may lead to unstable rates, he combined smaller ZIP codes, first using the spatial order method to determine the closeness of ZIP codes and then using a population threshold to determine how many ZIP codes close to each other should be combined.[17] He noted that this is an easier process when one is simply concerned about spatial proximity as a factor in combining ZIP code areas and not homogeneity of attributes (e.g., race, ethnicity, or socioeconomic status) in the resulting area.[17]

There are many studies that used the ZIP code to investigate pollution and health outcomes, often testing the hypothesis that people living in ZIP codes close to or containing a pollutant site have a larger burden of disease than those living in ZIP codes not close to or containing pollutant sites.[27,31] Baibergenova et al. used the ZIP code in this manner to investigate the relationship between proximity to waste sites contaminated with PCBs (polychlorinated biphenyls) and low birth weight in New York.[31] Clary and Ritz used this method to investigate the relationship between organochlorine pesticide exposure and pancreatic cancer.[27] Carpenter et al. counted ZIP codes by their distance from a pollution source and investigated endocrine disease in ZIP codes with and without Superfund sites.[24] Many of these studies cited the potential for error that comes with estimating an individual's exposure to a pollutant by using an exposure measure of a group, such as those residing in the same ZIP code; however, most noted that this error is most likely to lead to a decrease in sensitivity of the study and to bias the results toward the null, thereby underestimating individual exposure.[27,31] They cited benefits of ZIP code use, including the fact that they make investigations economical and may lead to hypothesis generation.[31]

ZIP codes have also been used for targeting public health interventions. Gordon et al., to target intervention, used the ZIP code of maternal residence to find regions experiencing high incidence rates of fetal malformations.[32] Stall et al. used the ZIP code to define study areas for an investigation of behaviors and cultures that promote high-risk behaviors such as alcohol and drug use, focusing on men who have sex with men (MSM) in four U.S. cities.[33] Luther et al. used ZIP codes to measure the impact of primary care programs directed toward reducing health disparities by coding ZIP codes as having either high or low access to primary care.[34] Benjamin and Platt used ZIP codes to decide to do targeted screening for lead in children.[35] Gould et al. used ZIP codes to identify areas with high birth rates among 15–17 year olds for purposes of targeting adolescent pregnancy prevention programs and concluded that the use of ZIP code-level data "holds promise for more effective program planning and intervention (p. 173)."[36] Banerjee and Carlin used the ZIP code to make smoothed maps of smoking cessation in southeastern Minnesota.[37]

ZIP codes have also been used in research investigating the connections between racial, ethnic, and socioeconomic characteristics and health outcomes, including elements of injustice and the notion of health disparities. One of the first investigations of environmental injustice, conducted by the United Church of Christ's Commission on Racial Justice in 1987, used ZIP codes to map the locations of hazardous facilities and the distribution of local populations according to racial, ethnic, and socioeconomic characteristics.[38] More recently, Wallace used ZIP codes to investigate different rates of decline of AIDS (acquired immunodeficiency syndrome) from 1993 to 1998 in New York City.[39] Feinglass et al. classified ZIP codes according to the proportion of population that is African American or low income to investigate whether rates of amputation and bypass surgery in northern Illinois were predicted by demographic information.[40] Philbin et al. investigated the impact of household income on the use of invasive procedures among patients with acute myocardial infarction.[41] The relationship between sociodemographic variables and unmarried teen childbirth was examined using the ZIP code for populations in California[42] and in Texas.[43] The relationship between environmental access to alcohol and resultant rates of both drinking and drinking and driving[44] as well as alcohol-related hospital admissions[45] has also been examined using the ZIP code as the geographic unit of analysis.

Finally, the ZIP code has been used in hospital discharge studies and the definition of health care-related geographic units. An example in Illinois is the work of the Chicago Department of Public Health on asthma hospital discharges in Chicago.[46] In addition, the Dartmouth Atlas of Health Care used a ZIP code boundary file obtained from a commercial firm, along with Medicare hospitalization records and the locations of acute care hospitals, to define hospital service areas based on the hospitals most used by local residents. Each ZIP code area was assigned to "the town containing the hospitals most often used by local residents (p. 13)," resulting in groups of ZIP codes assigned to a particular hospital service area. These areas were then visually examined to ensure that the ZIP code areas included in each service area were contiguous, and reassignment was performed when this was not the case. These areas were then used to map a variety of phenomena, such as Medicare reimbursements, the number of physicians in primary care, and the percentage of Medicare women undergoing a mammogram.[47] The *Dartmouth Atlas of Health Care* project continues, with several documents available for download from the *Dartmouth Atlas of Health Care* Web site (http://www.dartmouthatlas.org/index.shtm).

Similarly, ZIP codes were used to define utilization-based health care service areas called Primary Care Service Areas (PCSAs). Goodman et al. grouped 1999 U.S. ZIP codes into PCSAs based on where Medicare beneficiaries went to receive health care (i.e., the ZIP code where beneficiaries lived was assigned to the ZIP code of the provider that the plurality of beneficiaries visited). These areas were then adjusted based on geographic contiguity, population thresholds, and localization — "the degree to which primary care utilization occurred within PCSA boundaries (p. 290)."[48] The second version of PCSAs used ZCTAs instead of ZIP codes. Technical documentation describing the process of ZIP code and ZCTA assignment in detail is provided online by the Center for the Evaluative Clinical Sciences (CECS) at Dartmouth College on the Primary Care Service Area Project Web site (http://www.dartmouth.edu/~cecs/pcsa/pcsa.html). Boundary and data files for PCSAs are also available on the project Web site, as well as from the Health Resources and Services Administration (HRSA) Geospatial Data Warehouse (http://datawarehouse.hrsa.gov/pcsa.htm).

PCSAs have been used to map and analyze health-related phenomena. Mobley et al. used PCSAs to examine the relationship between demand factors (e.g., socioeconomic status, race); supply factors (e.g., access to physicians and other clinicians); intervening factors (e.g., travel times, urban/rural location, presence of managed care); and rates of hospital admissions of the elderly for ambulatory care sensitive conditions (ACSCs). They noted that PCSAs were chosen because they are assumed to be the "best approximation of the service areas in which the Medicare beneficiaries travel to receive ambulatory care, and are therefore the appropriate areal unit over which to construct aggregate rates for ACSC admissions."[49] The Marshfield clinic in Wisconsin has also delineated a health service area, the Marshfield Epidemiologic Study Area (MESA), built of 24 ZIP codes to facilitate study of health care utilization involving the clinic and its regional centers and affiliated hospitals.[50]

3.4 WORKING WITH ZIP CODES IN CANCER RESEARCH

When the choice is made to use the ZIP code as the geographic unit for cancer mapping and analysis, there are several key questions that must be addressed. How can the problem of spatial misalignment between the ZIP code and the ZCTA be addressed? Which single point location best represents a ZIP code area's population? How can this point be found and represented? This section addresses these questions.

3.4.1 ADDRESSING SPATIAL MISALIGNMENT

How can the problem of spatial misalignment between cancer data geocoded to the ZIP code and population data geocoded to the ZCTA or other areal unit be addressed?

If the researcher seeks to map the data using ZIP code boundaries, it is possible to impute populations for ZIP codes, provided an approximate ZIP code boundary file is available. There exist applications for interpolating sociodemographic information for units for which it is not collected (e.g., ZIP codes) from units for which it is (e.g., census tracts). The Long Island Areal Interpolator (http://gis.cancer.gov/nci/database. html#research) is one example of this type of application. In addition, approximate ZIP code boundaries, and population data, can be obtained from commercial firms, although the process of generating polygons to represent ZIP code service areas has been criticized for introducing representational error.[6] Grubesic and Matisziw developed a simple coefficient of ZIP code uncertainty (CZU_i) to measure the "local concentration of non-native street segments within a ZIP code area relative to the number of non-native segments for all ZIP codes" in New York state, noting that the index provides "a baseline measure of spatial uncertainty and potential representational error associated with each ZIP code."[6]

However, mapping using bounded units gives the impression that a phenomenon, such as a cancer rate, stops abruptly at the boundaries of the geographic unit; in reality, it is more likely to be a continuous phenomenon.[51] In addition, bounded units do not allow the researcher to control the spatial basis of support (e.g., the base population used in the calculation of disease rates) and thus are subject to statistical variation and instability. Stability in rates for bounded areas can be partially achieved through smoothing techniques, such as Bayesian adjustment.[52] Methods of density estimation or spatial filtering, especially adaptive filter density estimation, can be used to control the spatial basis of support from the outset as opposed to smoothing variation after it has already been mapped and result in a continuous surface map that is not subject to large amounts of statistical uncertainty.

In density estimation, a uniform grid is laid over the study area, and rates are calculated for each grid point by pulling in observations closest to that grid point, usually using a circular window.[53,54] In adaptive filter density estimation, the size of the circle used to calculate the rate expands until it pulls in a specified number of cases or a specified amount of population data.[54] For example, in constructing the map shown in Figure 3.1 of late-stage colorectal cancer in Iowa, a 3-mile grid was laid down over the state, and the indirectly adjusted proportion of late-stage cancer (i.e., late-stage colorectal cancers divided by all colorectal cancers) was calculated for each grid point using a circular window that expanded to pull in the closest 50 cases of colorectal cancer as aggregated by ZIP code. Figure 3.2 shows the filters used in calculating these rates in the Cedar Rapids, Iowa, area. Because of the spatial distribution of population density, filters in urban areas are smaller, and those in rural areas are larger.

The resulting rates of cancer calculated at each grid point can then be smoothed using inverse distance weighting and the eight nearest neighbors. Eight neighbors were chosen because this choice ensures that the smoothing of the data by the spatial filter is not again smoothed by a spatial smoothing function beyond the very local neighborhood of the grid.

Because adaptive filter density estimation makes use of spatial filters that expand until they have pulled in a threshold number of observations to achieve a stable rate calculation, the use of this method can partially overcome the problem of spatial

Colorectal Cancer Late Stage Rate, 1998-2003

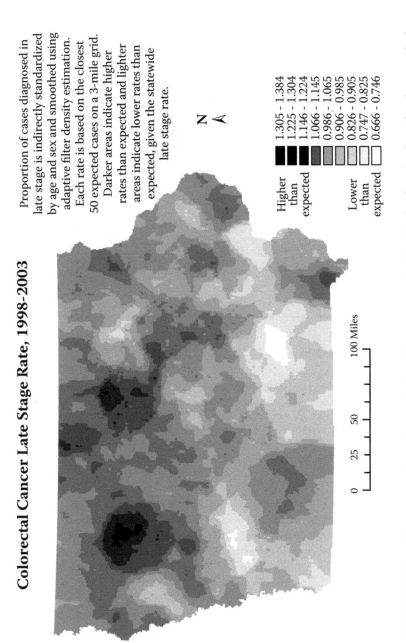

Proportion of cases diagnosed in late stage is indirectly standardized by age and sex and smoothed using adaptive filter density estimation. Each rate is based on the closest 50 expected cases on a 3-mile grid. Darker areas indicate higher rates than expected and lighter areas indicate lower rates than expected, given the statewide late stage rate.

Higher than expected
- 1.305 - 1.384
- 1.225 - 1.304
- 1.146 - 1.224
- 1.066 - 1.145
- 0.986 - 1.065
- 0.906 - 0.985
- 0.826 - 0.905
- 0.747 - 0.825
Lower than expected
- 0.666 - 0.746

0   25   50   100 Miles

FIGURE 3.1 Map of late-stage colorectal cancer in Iowa. Map was created using adaptive filter density estimation, a method that employs a filter of variable size to pull information in from estimated population center points containing cancer data aggregated by ZIP code to calculate a statistically stable indirectly standardized rate. (Cancer incidence data from the Iowa Cancer Registry.)

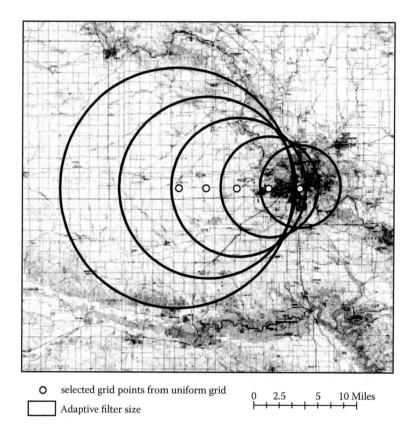

O   selected grid points from uniform grid

[   ] Adaptive filter size

0   2.5   5   10 Miles

FIGURE 3.2 The filters used to calculate the proportion of colorectal cancers diagnosed in the late stage for five grid points on a 3-mile grid in the Cedar Rapids, Iowa, area using adaptive filter density estimation. As demonstrated by the 1:100,000 topographic image, filters in urban areas are smaller, and those in rural areas are larger to pull in enough observations to calculate a stable rate. (Cancer incidence data from the Iowa Cancer Registry; 1:100,000 Digital Raster Graphic from the Iowa Geographic Image Map Server hosted by Iowa State University.)

misalignment between ZIP codes and ZCTAs. This is because the filter is basically a tool of spatial aggregation, pulling in data from neighboring ZIP codes, aggregating population and disease data for these ZIP codes and ZCTAs, and thus making a number of the borders drawn between ZCTAs meaningless in terms of separating population data. As much of the error in assigning population to ZCTAs likely occurs at the edges of contiguous ZIP code service areas, the error associated with the calculation of rates using density estimation is proportional to the number of ZCTA boundaries at the edges of the aggregated area. ZCTA boundaries that are drawn to either include population that should be associated with another ZIP code or exclude population that should be a part of the ZIP code in question will introduce error into the rate calculation. It is likely that error in rate calculation is greater in urban areas than in rural areas because fewer ZIP codes are pulled into the filters in urban areas, thus leaving more ZCTA borders "exposed." Figure 3.3 demonstrates

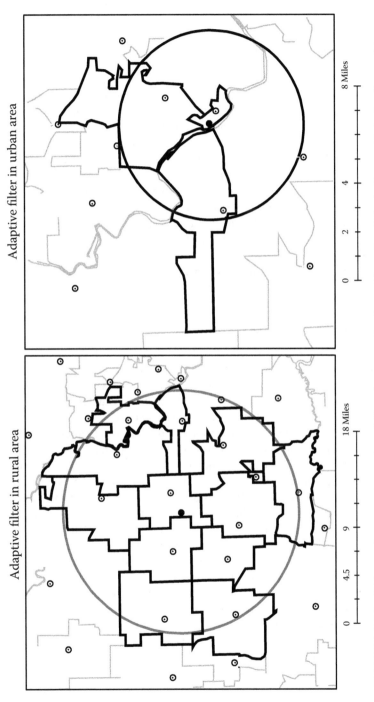

FIGURE 3.3 The difference between urban and rural filters in overcoming the problem of spatial misalignment between disease data geocoded to the ZIP code and population data geocoded to the ZCTA. The ZCTAs with bold lines are those pulled in by the adaptive filter and used in the rate calculation. A spatial filter in a rural area expands to pull in 13 ZIP codes/ZCTAs, thus combining data over a larger area and overcoming spatial misalignment in terms of the internal borders of the aggregated units; in an urban area, a spatial filter pulls in only 3 ZIP codes/ZCTAs, thus leaving more boundaries exposed. (Data from: Modified ZCTA boundaries, incorporated area polygons (not shown), and populated place locations from the Natural Resources GIS Library, hosted by the Iowa Department of Natural Resources and the U.S. Geological Survey; cancer incidence data from the Iowa Cancer Registry.)

the difference between urban and rural areas in terms of the proportion of ZCTA boundaries that are exposed. Although an urban filter pulls in only three ZIP codes/ZCTAs, a rural filter pulls in thirteen. The rural filter thus eliminates the problem of spatial misalignment in terms of the internal borders of the aggregated units. On the other hand, a larger proportion of the ZCTA borders are exposed in urban areas because fewer ZIP codes/ZCTAs are needed to achieve a stable rate calculation.

The problem of spatial misalignment in rate calculation using methods of density estimation could be entirely overcome if population data were tabulated and released by ZIP code instead of, or in addition to, tabulation and release by ZCTA. This is a simple matter as ZIP code information is collected during each census. In addition, a measure to indicate spatial uncertainty in population assignment could be developed for ZCTAs, similar to that developed by Grubesic and Matisziw for ZIP code areas. This type of measure could aid researchers in improving the accuracy of mapping and analysis. This would also be relatively straightforward as it is known how many addresses are associated with each ZIP code in each census block.[6,7]

To utilize this method, it is necessary to select a single point location to represent data obtained with the ZIP code as the geocode. This is also the case if the researcher seeks to calculate the distance between an individual and a health service when the only geocode available for the individual is the ZIP code.

3.4.2 FINDING A REPRESENTATIVE POINT LOCATION

Which single point location best represents the ZIP code? Efforts in the past have utilized the *centroid*, or geometric center, of a polygon for this purpose; this is problematic for two reasons. First, as the true boundaries of ZIP codes are not known, the polygons that would have to be used to calculate the centroid would be the ZCTA or the generalized ZIP code area polygons created by commercial firms. Second, there is no reason why the centroid of the polygon would be the most representative point when dealing with a phenomenon, such as late-stage colorectal cancer, that is directly linked to population. A more rational point to choose would be one that best represents the center of *population* in a ZIP code, not the center of land area.

A population center of a ZIP code ideally is defined as the location from which the sum of distances from all people in the ZIP code to itself is least. That is, if each person living in a ZIP code area made a trip to a location at its population center, both the total distance and the average distance would be shortest. Because the location of each individual in a ZIP code area is not known, we address other ways of approximating the location of this center. One interesting observation is that if any location in a ZIP code area contains more than half of the population of the ZIP code, it is the population center, as defined here, no matter where it is located. This is known as the *population median principle*.

How can this point representing the center of the population of a ZIP code be found? Two recently completed projects addressed this question. The first project enabled the mapping of breast, colorectal, and prostate cancer for the state of Iowa using adaptive filter density estimation and cancer data aggregated by ZIP code by using geographic and population information on census populated places and incorporated areas. The second project utilized free applications available on the Internet from Google®, Yahoo!® and other sources to geocode, map, and analyze residential locations of women seeking services at a women's health clinic to the post office representing their ZIP codes. We conclude with a discussion of another method for determining a point location that incorporates the use of census block population information, including demographic information such as the age and sex distribution of the population.

3.4.2.1 Cancer Mapping in Iowa Using ZIP-Coded Data

In this section, we trace the steps taken in producing detailed cancer maps from cancer registry data for which the finest-resolution geocodes are ZIP codes. As we intend to use density estimation, we start with the basic problem of defining the points that will best represent each ZIP code area. Because incorporated areas typically have locally significant populations, points representing centers of incorporated areas will often be population centers. We used publicly available geographic data sets — latitude and longitude coordinates of populated places, boundaries of incorporated areas, and ZCTA boundaries in Iowa — to identify estimated population center point locations for each ZIP code based on the above assumption. The ZIP code area boundaries used were derived directly from the ZCTA boundaries available on the U.S. Census Bureau Web site. The ZCTA boundary file was not used directly because some ZCTA codes represent several areas. All areas with the same ZCTA code were joined together so that there remained only one area for each ZCTA code, with 972 total areas, 949 of which are land based.

To find a representative point location for each ZCTA, we first limited our initial set of point locations (populated places) to those contained by incorporated area boundaries because it is likely that populated places within incorporated areas have higher populations than those located outside incorporated area boundaries. We then determined how many points fall in each land-based ZCTA. We divided the ZCTAs into three groups: those that contain only one point location, those that contain zero point locations, and those that contain multiple point locations. We determined which point to use as the estimated population center point for each ZCTA based on these groups (shown in Table 3.1). Where there was only one point, we used this point to represent the center of population as it was a location preferable to the ZCTA centroid. Where there were multiple points, we selected the point falling within the incorporated area with the highest population. Where there were zero points, we used the geometric center (centroid) of the ZCTA. In eight cases, a ZCTA contained multiple populated places, of which zero had available population data. In these cases, we chose to use the ZCTA centroid.

We visually compared the ZCTA centroids to our new set of estimated population center point locations. Figure 3.4 shows our comparison in central Iowa in terms of a base map of Iowa's topography (1:100,000 USGS digital raster graphic obtained from Iowa Geographic Map Server at http://ortho.gis.iastate.edu/). The borders shown are ZCTA boundaries, the white points represent ZCTA centroids, and the black points represent estimated population centers.

As a general trend, the estimated population center point seems to be a much more accurate geocode to use in representing the location of the concentration of the

TABLE 3.1

Assignment of Point Location to Represent ZCTA Population

Type of ZIP Code Tabulation Area (ZCTA)	Count	Type of Point Selected as ZIP Code Area Population Center
ZCTA contains only one populated place	753	We chose to use the populated place, and not the ZCTA centroid, as the populated place better represents the concentration of population within each ZIP code.
ZCTA contains zero populated places	78	We chose to use the ZCTA centroid to represent the population in these areas as no populated place is available.
ZCTA contains multiple populated places	110	We selected the populated place that represented the incorporated area with the highest 2000 population in each ZCTA.
ZCTA contains multiple populated places (none have population data)	8	We chose to use the ZCTA centroid to represent the population in these areas as no population information is available to use in choosing which populated area best represents the center of population.
Total ZCTAs	949	

Note: There were 23 water-based ZCTAs eliminated from the analysis as no population exists in these areas.

population in each area than the ZCTA centroid as ZCTA centroids are often located in uninhabited areas.

To evaluate the effectiveness of our method in identifying true ZIP code area population centers, we return to the idea of a population median (p-median). In keeping with the notion that any point representing more than half of the population of an area is the population median — the most representative location in an area in terms of population — we compared the populations of our estimated population centers with respect to total ZCTA populations to determine how many of our new points are population medians. To calculate these percentages, we first limited our data set to those ZCTAs for which we substituted the estimated population center point for the ZCTA centroid — the 753 ZCTAs containing one populated place and the 110 ZCTAs for which we chose the populated place contained within the highest populated incorporated area in the ZCTA — a total of 863 points.

In calculating the percentages of population represented at each point, we used incorporated area populations as the population of each populated place of the same name. As some populated places did not have population data (as they represented,

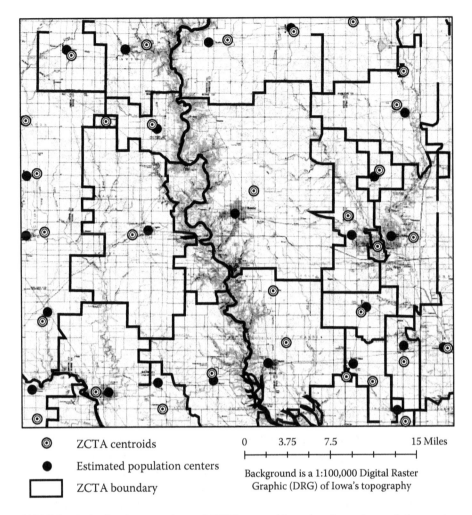

ZCTA centroids

Estimated population centers

ZCTA boundary

0   3.75   7.5   15 Miles

Background is a 1:100,000 Digital Raster
Graphic (DRG) of Iowa's topography

FIGURE 3.4 A visual comparison of ZCTA centroids and estimated population center points with respect to a base map of Iowa's topography. This demonstrates that estimated population center points are more accurate in representing the location of population within a ZIP code.

for example, a small place within a large incorporated area represented at a different location by a populated place), we removed all ZCTAs for which the estimated population center point contained no population — 11 records located in urban areas. Also, as some incorporated areas cover more land area than the ZCTA in which the populated place representing that incorporated area is contained, some of our estimated population center points had more population than the ZCTA that contained them; we removed all ZCTAs for which the estimated population center point had more than 100% of the ZCTA population — 71 records located primarily in urban areas and in very small rural ZCTAs. We were left with a set of 781 point locations.

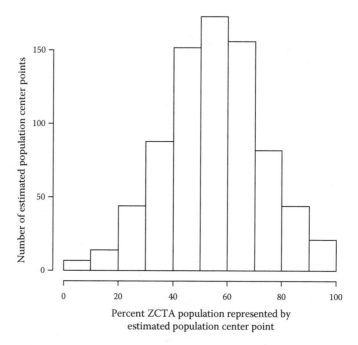

FIGURE 3.5 The distribution of estimated population center points with respect to the percentage of the ZCTA population with their respective incorporated areas represented.

Figure 3.5 shows the distribution of estimated population centers regarding the percentage of the ZCTA population they represent. On average, the estimated population center points represent approximately 55% of the ZCTA population. A total of 476 (60.9%) estimated population centers represented 50% or more of their respective ZCTA populations. Recall that these points represent ZCTAs of two types: those that contained only one point and those that contained multiple points. When we examine the distribution of estimated population centers regarding percentage of the ZCTA population represented, broken down by these two categories as shown in Figure 3.6, we see that ZCTAs containing multiple points (from which we chose the highest populated point) were more likely to represent 50% or greater of the ZCTA population than those for which there was only one point. The proportion of estimated centers that represented 50% or more of their ZCTA populations was 67.0% for ZCTAs with multiple incorporated areas and 60.7% for ZCTAs for which there was only one incorporated area. This may indicate that the very rural ZCTAs, containing only one incorporated area, may have a more dispersed population that is more difficult to represent at a single point than those ZCTAs that are more urban and contain multiple incorporated areas. Table 3.2 shows information about the distributions of estimated population center points.

In addition, as shown in Figure 3.7, the percentage of the population represented at an estimated population center correlates positively with the size of the ZCTA population (.308) and the size of the incorporated area population (.468).

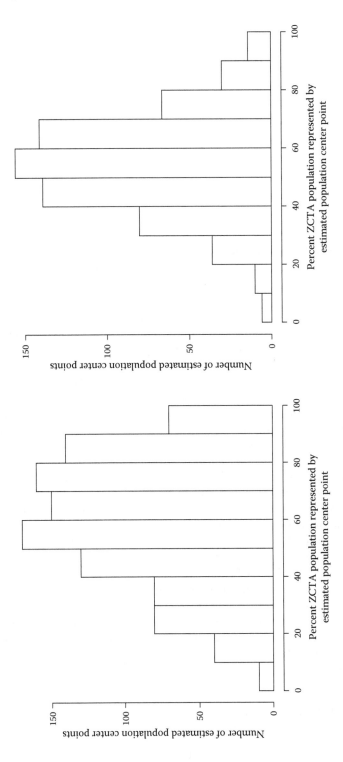

FIGURE 3.6 The distribution shown in Figure 3.5 is broken down by the two types of ZCTAs, those that contain multiple incorporated areas (left) and those that contain only one incorporated area (right).

TABLE 3.2

Descriptive Statistics for the Distributions of Estimated Population Center Points

	Min	Max	Mean	Median	SD	Skewness	Kurtosis	≥50%
All ZCTAs	0.2	99.6	54.9	54.9	17.8	−0.1	−0.01	60.9
Multiple center ZCTAs	1.1	99.6	59.1	61.1	22.1	−0.3	−0.49	67.0
Single center ZCTAs	0.2	99.4	54.2	54.2	17.0	−0.1	0.07	60.7

These correlations differ for the two types of ZCTAs. The correlations between percentage of the population represented and ZCTA population and percentage of the population represented and incorporated area population were .433 and .659 for ZCTAs with multiple incorporated areas and .254 and .424 for ZCTAs with a single incorporated area, respectively. In other words, ZCTAs with higher populations and incorporated areas with higher populations also had higher percentages of the population covered by the estimated population center point. Geographic information system (GIS) operations were performed with ArcMap™ software, and statistical analyses were performed using R, an open source statistical program.[55]

Overall, this method was based on sound theoretical grounds, was fairly easy and fast to implement, and utilized publicly available data. However, it was limited because we chose to use geometric centers (centroids) of ZCTAs as our point locations in ZCTAs that included zero populated places or multiple populated places for which no population data were available. A better method would incorporate the use of population distribution information within these ZCTAs as well. The p-median calculations indicate that our method may result in the most improvement in representing population in more urban areas. As a number of the records had to be removed from the analysis because of lack of population data or very large incorporated areas that extended beyond ZCTA boundaries and contained more population than the ZCTAs located in urban areas, it is likely that our method is most effective in midsize, semiurban ZIP code areas, those with multiple incorporated areas that are not very large metropolitan areas but are also not so rural that they have an insignificant concentration of population in one incorporated area and a population that is more dispersed throughout the ZCTA. Although we were unable to calculate percentage of the population represented in all ZCTAs, the visual comparison of ZCTA centroids to estimated population centers regarding topography indicates that our method, although subject to limitations, represents an improvement over the use of ZCTA centroids.

3.4.2.2 The Post Office as Geocode

Post office locations offer a reasonable estimate of the population center for ZIP codes in the United States (i.e., the hypothetical center of population for all those

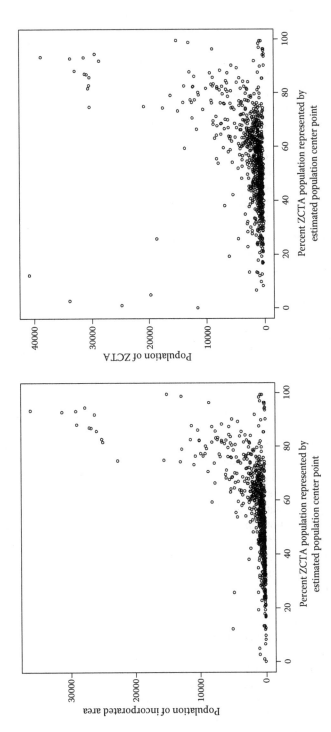

FIGURE 3.7 The correlation between the percentage of the population represented by the estimated population center point and the incorporated area population (left) and the correlation between the percentage of the population represented by the estimated population center point and the total ZCTA population (right).

with the same ZIP code) largely because of the unique business model utilized by the USPS that governs office placement. More specifically, the basis for taking advantage of post offices for such a purpose lies in the Congressional mandate given to the USPS under the Postal Reorganization Act of 1971 to offer "a fundamental service" to the American people on a "fair and equitable basis."[56] The USPS operationalizes this mandate by providing home delivery service to every residence in the country as efficiently and cost-effectively as possible, which they refer to as "universal service."[56] For the purpose of estimating ZIP code population centers, this has important implications, which are explored here.

Not only must a post office be located within a short daily travel distance of all residents served on its delivery routes, but also it must be centrally located within the population so that services only available at physical locations can be accessed as equitably as possible by all customers — also a part of what USPS considers universal service.[56] This has led to the expansion of convenience — or storefront — locations that do not serve the traditional dual role of base for delivery routes and service location but instead are meant only to broaden storefront service access. For all of these reasons and in the absence of a gold standard method, post offices can be used as an adequate estimate of ZIP code population centers.

Post offices were used to estimate population centers during the development of a geocoding protocol for a proposed research project, Intimate Partner Violence in Women Seeking Abortive Services.[57] As it would be most efficient to have those delivering mail drive the shortest distance to make their deliveries, doing so from a post office located at the population center of their delivery area most efficiently achieves this end. Indeed, even in 1971 when the Postal Reorganization Act was passed, universal service was not a nascent mission of the USPS. This service goal actually has a history stretching back to the beginnings of the postal service, making it an ingrained and indispensable part of our communities.[58]

The proposed study called for the development of a protocol that allowed geographic analysis, using only ZIP codes, of study participants with respect to their estimated home locations and available community intimate partner violence (IPV) resources. This analysis was also intended for comparison of reported rates of IPV to aspects of geography in relation to risk. The vulnerable status of the planned study population (those seeking abortions) as well as the IPV resources mapped (many of which were domestic violence shelters) prevented further specification beyond the ZIP code level (or in the case of some resources, their post office box locations). The use of post office geocodes provided a balance between security and analysis by maintaining a certain level of confidentiality for participants while still differentiating latitudes and longitudes enough to offer insight into how location affects access to resources and experience with IPV.

Justifying the use of post offices as an appropriate population centroid estimate was only the first step in the ultimate aim of obtaining the best possible geocode for given ZIP codes. The next task was to evaluate the feasibility of obtaining and processing information on post offices statewide in Iowa, which appeared potentially daunting considering that nationally there are over 42,000 ZIP codes serviced by the USPS and roughly 37,000 post offices. The task proved practicable, however, when it was found that the total number of ZIP codes in Iowa around the time of the U.S.

Census Bureau's creation of ZCTAs (i.e., 1999) was 1073. During the 2000 census, 949 land-based ZCTAs were created for the same area, providing standardized geographic boundaries for ZIP codes but reducing the original total by 124 (11.6%).

A simple request to the USPS for a comprehensive list of all post offices in Iowa, including expansion branches and storefront locations, turned up 891 locations.[59] However, after this list was cross-checked with a large online address and phone directory, [30] more post office locations were identified and added (excluding locations serving only distribution and administrative purposes), for a final total of 921 locations.[60] For the purposes of the protocol, the number of post offices compared favorably to the 1073 ZIP codes listed for Iowa — an almost one-to-one ratio. Ultimately, the existence of 85.8% as many post offices as ZIP codes and 97.1% as many ZCTAs as post offices helps to demonstrate the high level of population-specific service provided by the USPS in Iowa, despite the small ratio of human population to land mass in the state.

The final protocol for the study was successfully tested using a pilot population from the future clinical survey site. Table 3.3 gives frequencies and percentages for the steps involved in protocol development. The geocoding, population center estimations, GIS mapping, and straight-line distance calculations were all performed using freely available Internet resources, including the Google Earth™ mapping service, Yahoo!® Maps API (application programming interface), Batchgeocode.com,

TABLE 3.3
Pilot Record Frequencies for Protocol Steps

	Frequency (n/total n)	Percentage (%)
Total number of post offices geocoded by address	921/921	100.0
Total number of pilot record ZIP codes[a] geocoded to the geographic centroid of the ZCTA	229/1083	21.1
Geographic centroids of the ZCTA reassigned to estimated population centers (i.e., post office/ branch locations)	167/229	72.9
Total number of intimate partner violence (IPV) resources geocoded by exact address	21/44	47.7
Total number of IPV resource locations estimated by local post office/branch location	22/44	50.0
Total number of pilot records weighted[b] to accurately reflect those with repeated (nonunique) ZIP codes for help with later analyses of geographic resource access	229/1083	21.1
Total number of straight-line distance estimates obtained between 1083 pilot records and 43 IPV resources	9847/9847	100.0

[a] Not all pilot records had their own unique ZIP code; many were repeated.
[b] Each repeated ZIP code was multiplied according to the number of records reporting it.

and a Microsoft Excel® software-based geocoding program from Juice Analytics® software.[61–64] The use of freely available resources was part of an intentional effort to keep costs down while reducing the need for high levels of technical expertise.

We began our process by compiling a comprehensive list of all post offices as described (including addresses) located within any of the potential ZIP codes that study participants might report as their home locations. A comprehensive list of all ZIP codes and ZCTAs for the state, available from the USPS and the U.S. Census Bureau, respectively, then needed to be obtained.[58,65,66] Finally, a list of IPV resources and addresses had to be compiled. The lists of post offices and ZIP codes were then compared, and any ZIP codes not containing a post office were noted. Finally, the list of pilot record ZIP codes was scrutinized for duplicates to arrive at the actual number of unique ZIP codes to be geocoded. The geocoding of only unique pilot record ZIP codes meant that geocodes had to be weighted retrospectively according to how many pilot records each actually represented. Weighting of ZIP codes was necessary for accurate analyses of geographic access because of the high rate of pilot records containing the same ZIP codes.

All of the collected addresses and unique ZIP codes were imported into a Microsoft Excel software-based program for geocoding. The program feeds the data through an Internet connection to the Yahoo! Maps API for geocoding of both addresses and ZIP codes with a daily maximum of 5000 locations. The program returns latitude and longitude coordinates for all entries based on near-exact locations for addresses and geographic centroid estimates of corresponding ZCTAs (through interpolation) for ZIP codes. The addressed-based geocodes, as well as geocodes from ZIP codes that were determined not to have a post office listed and geocodes based on post office boxes of resource sites, could then be considered final, but geocodes within a ZCTA containing a post office still had to be adjusted. Adjustments were performed using a spreadsheet program to replace the geocodes for the ZCTA geographic centroids with the geocodes for the post offices in that ZCTA. Again, pilot records within ZIP codes lacking a post office were excluded from the adjustment process after a geographic centroid had been obtained for the ZIP code.

Once all of the information had been geocoded and adjusted, Juice Analytics Excel Geocoding Tool, V2™ was utilized to create a Keyhole™ map layer (KML) file to be displayed in the free GIS mapping program Google Earth.[62,63] The accuracy of the Excel Geocoding Tool is comparable to that of any commercially available GIS mapping tool, such as those commonly used in vehicle and mobile phone navigation systems.[64] Figure 3.8 gives a graphic example of the effect of the ZCTA centroid to post office location adjustment by showing the difference between the two locations with respect to population density and topography.[67]

Information on centroid adjustment and access statistics was obtained using Batchgeocode.com and by weighting of the pilot records.[61,64] For the entire sample of pilot records with unique ZIP codes ($n = 229$), the average travel distance of each adjustment was 1.4 miles. After weighting of each ZIP code according to the corresponding pilot records containing that ZIP code, the average minimum straight-line distance to the first IPV resource for the entire sample ($n = 1083$) was 6.60 miles, with a range of 0.02 to 47.20 miles. In addition, the weighted average straight-line

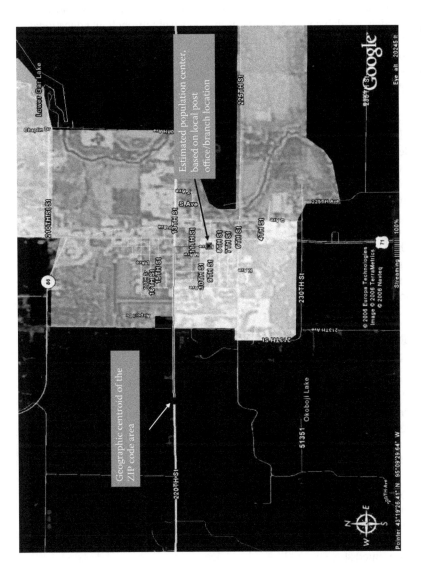

FIGURE 3.8 The geographic centroid to estimated population center adjustment (based on post office location) in Milford, Iowa. Lighter colors indicate higher population density (e.g., white is 800+ people per square mile). Darker colors represent lower population density (translucent black is 2 or fewer people per square mile).[62,67] (Photo from Google Earth™ mapping service. With permission.)

distance between pilot records and the clinic study site, where pilot records were obtained, was 28.08 miles, with a range of 1.06 to 168.53 miles.

Overall, advantages of this approach lie in its comprehensibility and accessibility to users otherwise unfamiliar with geocoding and GIS mapping applications. ZIP codes and the post offices that serve them are ubiquitous in America and universally familiar. Likewise, Microsoft Office® software, including the Excel spreadsheet program, is widely available and currently used extensively throughout educational settings and the allied health fields. Finally, expansion of what is possible through Internet resources is likely to continue, making increasingly complex analyses, such as batch calculation of routing information (i.e., travel distance and time variously known as proximity analysis or network analysis) between two geocodes, possible. All of these factors combine to make the approach appealing.

Regionally, the advantages of using post offices as geocodes can vary, as there are many differences in the numbers of ZIP codes used per state, population density per ZIP code, and the number of ZIP codes served by a single post office. All of these factors can change the level of improvement achieved by substituting post office-based population center estimates for ZCTA centroids. Finally, a disadvantage of the method is that it seems an unlikely candidate for becoming the eventual gold standard as the basis for its use relies heavily on the ability of the USPS to fulfill its congressional mandate successfully and not on more objective measures of population location such as census data. In the more densely populated parts of the country with above-average real estate and rental prices, universal storefront access can become nearly impossible because of cost — implying greater usefulness for this technique in rural states such as Iowa, where cost is less likely to impede such access.

3.4.3 USING CENSUS BLOCK POPULATION DATA TO FIND THE POPULATION-WEIGHTED ZIP CODE CENTER

When the researcher has access only to the ZIP code and seeks to determine the best location within the ZIP code to represent the population, one can also take advantage of population data by census block, which is the smallest areal unit for which population data are tabulated by the U.S. Census Bureau. ZCTAs, which as described are generalized representations of ZIP code areas, are built of census blocks. The population of each census block can be used as weights in determining where to locate an estimated population center point. In addition, if information on the age, sex, race, and ethnicity of the individuals living in each block can also be obtained, researchers can use this information to find estimated population centers that are weighted by these demographic variables (e.g., the estimated Hispanic population center or the estimated age 65+ population center) to support analyses concerning particular communities of interest.

A simple example of a method that has been used in the literature[54] for determining an estimated population center of a ZIP code using block population weights follows. We start with the latitude and longitude coordinates for the centroids of each block within a ZCTA. As we are dealing with two-dimensional space, we can find the mean latitude and mean longitude values, which will yield the coordinates of the mean geometric location. This gives us the point for which the sum of the squared distances from all of the latitude

TABLE 3.4

Method Incorporating Block Populations to Find Population-Weighted ZIP Code Center

Block ID b	Longitude x	Latitude y	Population p	Weighted longitude yw = y*p	Weighted latitude xw = x*p
1	−94.9299	44.7668	613	−58,192.0247	27,442.0702
2	−95.0868	44.2438	570	−54,199.4931	25,218.9557
3	−95.3860	44.5941	671	−64,003.9766	29,922.6084
4	−95.3872	43.7945	553	−52,749.1453	24,218.3495
5	−95.4006	43.5915	697	−66,494.2162	30,383.2609
6	−95.6505	44.0099	636	−60,833.7052	27,990.3085
7	−95.7801	44.5545	545	−52,200.1511	24,282.2121
8	−96.1221	44.8341	683	−65,651.3759	30,621.6889
9	−95.8712	44.8652	685	−65,671.7968	30,732.6946
10	−95.1683	44.3955	642	−61,098.0624	28,501.9191
Total			6295	−601,093.9473	279,314.0680
Mean				−95.4875	44.3708

and longitude coordinates to itself is least. To weight this by population, we take into account the populations of the blocks that are aggregated to build the ZCTA. Although the final estimated population center point will be affected by the aggregation of population data to block centroids, this is the only way to proceed when the finest-resolution population data available are aggregated by block centroid. We obtain population counts for each block; when we are interested in a particular demographic group, we would instead obtain the population of that particular group. We then multiply the latitude and longitude coordinates for each block centroid by the population of the block, resulting in weighted latitude and longitude values. We sum these weighted latitude and longitude values and divide each sum by the total population of the ZCTA. Table 3.4 shows a hypothetical set of locations and populations and gives the resultant calculations as well as the final weighted mean latitude and longitude coordinates.

This process could also be done using the median instead of the mean, although it is a more complicated computation. A similar method of population weighting using block populations can be used to find the most likely distance an individual must travel to a particular health service when only the ZIP code of the individual is known.

3.5 CONCLUSION

Despite the limitations of the ZIP code, its use in cancer prevention and control research and practice is likely to grow because it is widely available and representative of a relatively small geographic area. Because of these advantages, researchers are finding ways to overcome its major limitations. Mapping using bounded areas is problematic as it fails to adequately control the spatial basis of support and can mislead the map reader. No areal unit is perfect, and researchers must become familiar with the strengths and limitations of any unit chosen. Also, as noted, it is critical to understand the scale at which a process operates as the use of different geographic units will result in different patterns. Choosing a unit appropriate to the scale of the phenomenon in question is a primary concern. In addition, the choice to use the ZIP code has implications for spatial analyses such as cluster detection. Grubesic and Matisziw found that the choice of areal unit to use in representing the ZIP code (i.e., a ZIP code polygon created by a commercial firm or a ZCTA polygon created by the U.S. Census Bureau) can affect the identification of cancer clusters generated using Moran's I statistic (a local measure of spatial autocorrelation) as the bounding and spatial extent of these two types of units differ.[6]

There is likely to be an increase in the use of methods, such as density estimation and spatial filtering, that seek to control the spatial basis of support and avoid or overcome the problems posed by bounded units. When using these methods to study aggregated data, often the only type of data available because of privacy concerns, it becomes necessary to choose a point location to which population and health data can be attached. This is also the case when seeking to calculate the distance between individuals and a health service when the only geocode available for the individual is the ZIP code. The choice of a point location that represents the population of an area, or an individual for whom the only available geocode is the ZIP code, is a choice that should not be made lightly, especially when the choice will affect the resulting map or distance calculations made from an individual to a health facility.

The best protocols to follow in data collection and tabulation should be a subject of discussion as the choice of how to collect and tabulate data, and what to make available to the public, governs the ability of researchers and practitioners to investigate the geographical patterns of cancer and to most effectively target prevention and control efforts geographically.

REFERENCES

1. Willis, A.; Krewski, D.; Jerrett, M.; Goldberg, M. S.; Burnett, R. T. Selection of ecologic covariates in the American Cancer Society study. *J Toxicol Environ Health A* 2003, 66, 1563–89.
2. U.S. Census Bureau. Glossary of terms for the economic census. http://help.econ. census.gov/econhelp/glossary/. (accessed December 6, 2006)
3. U.S. Census Bureau answers to frequently asked questions about census bureau geography. Maps and mapping engines: ZIP code information. http://www.census. gov/geo/www/tiger/tigermap.html#ZIP. (accessed December 6, 2006)
4. Johnson, G. D. Small area mapping of prostate cancer incidence in New York State (USA) using fully Bayesian hierarchical modelling. *Int J Health Geogr* 2004, 3, 29.
5. Jacquez, G. M.; Greiling, D. A. Local clustering in breast, lung and colorectal cancer in Long Island, New York. *Int J Health Geogr* 2003, 2, 3.
6. Grubesic, T. H.; Matisziw, T. C. On the use of ZIP codes and ZIP Code Tabulation Areas (ZCTAs) for the spatial analysis of epidemiological data. *Int J Health Geogr* 2006, 5, 58.

7. U.S. Census Bureau ZIP Code® Tabulation Areas (ZCTAs™). http://www.census.gov/ geo/ZCTA/zcta.html. (accessed December 7, 2006)

8. Carretta, H. J.; Mick, S. S. Geocoding public health data. *Am J Public Health* 2003, 93, 699; author reply 699–700.

9. Krieger, N.; Waterman, P.; Chen, J. T.; Soobader, M. J.; Subramanian, S. V.; Carson, R. Krieger et al. respond. *Am J Public Health* 2003, 93, 699–700.

10. Krieger, N.; Waterman, P.; Chen, J. T.; Soobader, M. J.; Subramanian, S. V.; Carson, R. ZIP code caveat: bias due to spatiotemporal mismatches between ZIP codes and U.S. census-defined geographic areas — the Public Health Disparities Geocoding Project. *Am J Public Health* 2002, 92, 1100–2.

11. Krieger, N.; Chen, J. T.; Waterman, P. D.; Soobader, M. J.; Subramanian, S. V.; Carson, R. Geocoding and monitoring of U.S. socioeconomic inequalities in mortality and cancer incidence: does the choice of area-based measure and geographic level matter? The Public Health Disparities Geocoding Project. *Am J Epidemiol* 2002, 156, 471–82.

12. U.S. Census Bureau Census 2000 data for the state of Iowa. http://www.census.gov/ census2000/states/ia.html. (accessed November 12, 2006)

13. U.S. Census Bureau Iowa census data tables: ZIP Code Tabulation Areas. http://data. iowadatacenter.org/browse/ZCTAs.html. (accessed November 11, 2006)

14. U.S. Census Bureau Census 2000 — summary data profiles: ZCTAs. http://www.nyloves-biz.com/nysdc/census2000/2KZCTAProfiles.asp. (accessed November 11, 2006)

15. U.S. Census Bureau Census 2000 data for the state of New York. http://www.census. gov/census2000/states/ny.html. (accessed November 13, 2006)

16. Thomas, A. J.; Eberly, L. E.; Smith, G. D.; Neaton, J. D. ZIP-code-based versus tract-based income measures as long-term risk-adjusted mortality predictors. *Am J Epidemiol* 2006, 164, 6, 586–590.

17. Wang, F. Spatial clusters of cancers in Illinois 1986–2000. *J Med Syst* 2004, 28, 237–56.

18. Diez-Roux, A. V. Investigating neighborhood and area effects on health. *Am J Public Health* 2001, 91, 1783–89.

19. Diez-Roux, A. V. Invited commentary: places, people and health. *Am J Epidemiol* 2002, 155, 516–19.

20. Olson, D. ZIP codes and census tracts in the Iowa Cancer Registry. In *A Short Note on ZIP Code and Census Tract Completeness and Accuracy as Geocodes in the Iowa Cancer Registry*, personal communication, Iowa City, Iowa, 2006.

21. Office for Civil Rights. Summary of the HIPAA Privacy Rule. U.S. Department of Health and Human Services. http:// www.hhs.gov/ocr/hipaa/ (accessed December 4, 2006)

22. National Institutes of Health. Protecting Personal Health Information in Research: Understanding the HIPAA Privacy Rule. U.S. Department of Health and Human Services. http://privacyruleandresearch.nih.gov/pr_02.asp. (accessed December 13, 2006)

23. National Institutes of Health. HIPAA Privacy Rule for Researchers. U.S. Department of Health and Human Services. http://privacyruleandresearch.nih.gov/ (accessed December 4, 2006)

24. Carpenter, D. O.; Shen, Y.; Nguyen, T.; Le, L.; Lininger, L. L. Incidence of endocrine disease among residents of New York areas of concern. *Environ Health Perspect* 2001, 109 Suppl 6, 845–51.

25. Jacquez, G. M.; Greiling, D. A. Geographic boundaries in breast, lung and colorectal cancers in relation to exposure to air toxics in Long Island, New York. *Int J Health Geogr* 2003, 2, 4.

26. Goovaerts, P.; Jacquez, G. M. Accounting for regional background and population size in the detection of spatial clusters and outliers using geostatistical filtering and spatial neutral models: the case of lung cancer in Long Island, New York. *Int J Health Geogr* 2004, 3, 14.

27. Clary, T.; Ritz, B. Pancreatic cancer mortality and organochlorine pesticide exposure in California, 1989–1996. *Am J Ind Med* 2003, 43, 306–13.

28. White, E.; Aldrich, T. E. Geographic studies of pediatric cancer near hazardous waste sites. *Arch Environ Health* 1999, 54, (6), 390–397.

29. McGinnis, L. S.; Menck, H. R.; Eyre, H. J.; Bland, K. I.; Scott-Conner, C. E.; Morrow, M.; Winchester, D. P. National Cancer Data Base survey of breast cancer management for patients from low income ZIP codes. *Cancer* 2000, 88, 933–45.

30. Nash, D.; Azeez, S.; Vlahov, D.; Schori, M. Evaluation of an intervention to increase screening colonoscopy in an urban public hospital setting. *J Urban Health* 2006, 83, 2, 231–243.

31. Baibergenova, A.; Kudyakov, R.; Zdeb, M.; Carpenter, D. O. Low birth weight and residential proximity to PCB-contaminated waste sites. *Environ Health Perspect* 2003, 111, 1352–57.

32. Gordon, T. E.; Leeth, E. A.; Nowinski, C. J.; MacGregor, S. N.; Kambich, M.; Silver, R. K. Geographic and temporal analysis of folate-sensitive fetal malformations. *J Soc Gynecol Invest* 2003, 10, 298–301.

33. Stall, R.; Paul, J. P.; Greenwood, G.; Pollack, L. M.; Bein, E.; Crosby, G. M.; Mills, T. C.; Binson, D.; Coates, T. J.; Catania, J. A. Alcohol use, drug use and alcohol-related problems among men who have sex with men: the Urban Men's Health Study. *Addiction* 2001, 96, 1589–1601.

34. Luther, S. L.; Studnicki, J.; Kromrey, J.; Lomando-Frakes, K.; Grant, P.; Finley, G. C. A method to measure the impact of primary care programs targeted to reduce racial and ethnic disparities in health outcomes. *J Public Health Manag Pract* 2003, 9, 243–48.

35. Benjamin, J. T.; Platt, C. Is universal screening for lead in children indicated? An analysis of lead results in Augusta, Georgia in 1997. *J Med Assoc Ga* 1999, 88, 24–26.

36. Gould, J. B.; Herrchen, B.; Pham, T.; Bera, S.; Brindis, C. Small-area analysis: targeting high-risk areas for adolescent pregnancy prevention programs. *Fam Plann Perspect* 1998, 30, 173–76.

37. Banerjee, S.; Carlin, B. P. Parametric spatial cure rate models for interval-censored time-to-relapse data. *Biometrics* 2004, 60, 268–75.

38. Maantay, J. Mapping environmental injustices: pitfalls and potential of geographic information systems in assessing environmental health and equity. *Environ Health Perspect* 2002, 110 Suppl 2, 161–71.

39. Wallace, R. G. AIDS in the HAART era: New York's heterogeneous geography. *Soc Sci Med* 2003, 56, 1155–71.

40. Feinglass, J.; Kaushik, S.; Handel, D.; Kosifas, A.; Martin, G. J.; Pearce, W. H. Peripheral bypass surgery and amputation: northern Illinois demographics, 1993 to 1997. *Arch Surg* 2000, 135, 75–80.

41. Philbin, E. F.; McCullough, P. A.; DiSalvo, T. G.; Dec, G. W.; Jenkins, P. L.; Weaver, W. D. Socioeconomic status is an important determinant of the use of invasive procedures after acute myocardial infarction in New York State. *Circulation* 2000, 102 (19 Suppl 3), III107–15.

42. Kirby, D.; Coyle, K.; Gould, J. B. Manifestations of poverty and birthrates among young teenagers in California ZIP code areas. *Fam Plann Perspect* 2001, 33, 63–69.

43. Blake, B. J.; Bentov, L. Geographical mapping of unmarried teen births and selected sociodemographic variables. *Public Health Nurs* 2001, 18, 33–39.

44. Gruenewald, P. J.; Johnson, F. W.; Treno, A. J. Outlets, drinking and driving: a multilevel analysis of availability. *J Stud Alcohol* 2002, 63, 460–68.
45. Tatlow, J. R.; Clapp, J. D.; Hohman, M. M. The relationship between the geographic density of alcohol outlets and alcohol-related hospital admissions in San Diego County. *J Community Health* 2000, 25, 79–88.
46. Dobbs, D. J.; Lanum, A.; Thomas, S. D. *Asthma Hospital Discharges in Chicago — Racial Disparity.* Epidemiology Program, Chicago Department of Public Health, Chicago, 2004.
47. The Center for the Evaluative Clinical Sciences, Dartmouth Medical School. *The Dartmouth Atlas of Health Care in the United States.* American Hospital Publishing, Chicago, 1996.
48. Goodman, D. C.; Mick, S. S.; Bott, D.; Stukel, T.; Chang, C. H.; Marth, N.; Poage, J.; Carretta, H. J. Primary care service areas: a new tool for the evaluation of primary care services. *Health Serv Res* 2003, 38 (1 Pt 1), 287–309.
49. Mobley, L. R.; Root, E.; Anselin, L.; Lozano-Gracia, N.; Koschinsky, J. Spatial analysis of elderly access to primary care services. *Int J Health Geogr* 2006, 5, 19.
50. Marshfield Clinic Research Foundation, Marshfield Epidemiologic Study Area. http://www.marshfieldclinic.org/merc/pages/default.aspx?page=mcrf_merc_study_mesa (accessed October 30, 2006)
51. Rushton, G. Public health, GIS, and spatial analytic tools. *Annu Rev Public Health* 2003, 24, 43–56.
52. Bithell, J. A classification of disease mapping methods. *Stat Med* 2000, 19, 2203–15.
53. Rushton, G.; Lolonis, P. Exploratory spatial analysis of birth defect rates in an urban population. *Stat Med* 1996, 15, 717–26.
54. Talbot, T. O.; Kulldorff, M.; Forand, S. P.; Haley, V. B. Evaluation of spatial filters to create smoothed maps of health data. *Stat Med* 2000, 19, 2399–2408.
55. Team, R. D. C. *R: A Language and Environment for Statistical Computing.* R Foundation for Statistical Computing, Vienna, Austria, 2006.
56. *United States Postal Service Annual Report* 2005. U.S. Postal Service, Washington, DC, 2005, p. 26. http://www.usps.com/history/anrpt05/ (accessed August 8, 2006)
57. Saftlas, A. F. Intimate partner violence in women seeking abortive services. Unpublished protocol.University of Iowa, Iowa City, 2006.
58. *The United States Postal Service: An American History* 1775–2002. United States Postal Service, Washington, DC, 2003. pp. 36–37. http://www.usps.com/cpim/ftp/pubs/pub100/.pdf (accessed August 8, 2006)
59. Rose, D. USPS Business Service Network. Personal Communication, 2006.
60. Switchboard.com: Your Digital Directory. InfoSpace, Inc. http://www.switchboard.com (accessed April 1, 2006)
61. Yahoo! Developer Network. http://developer.yahoo.com/maps/simple/index.html (April 1).
62. *Google Earth,*™ version 3.0.0762. Google Software, Mountain View, CA, 2005.
63. Juice Analytics. *Excel Geocoding Tool,* version 2. Juice Analytics, Herndon, VA, 2006.
64. Holmstrand, P. Batchgeocode.com: Map multiple locations/find address coordinates. http://www.batchgeocode.com (accessed April 26, 2006)
65. U.S. Census Bureau Census 2000 U.S. Gazetteer files. http://www.census.gov/geo/www/gazetteer/places2k.html (accessed November 11, 2006)
66. Address Information Systems (AIS) Products. http://www.usps.com/ncsc/addressinfo/addressinfomenu.htm (accessed November 11, 2006)
67. Juice Analytics. *Population Density by County and by Census Blocks.* Juice Analytics, Herndon, VA, 2006.

4 Producing Spatially Continuous Prostate Cancer Maps with Different Geocodes and Spatial Filter Methods

Gerard Rushton, Qiang Cai, and Zunqiu Chen

CONTENTS

4.1 INTRODUCTION

Spatially continuous cancer maps can be designed to convey more realistically spatial patterns of cancer, yet they are rarely used. In this chapter, we discuss the relative merits of two different methods, upscaling and downscaling, for producing such maps. Using geocoded prostate cancer incidence stage records from a cancer registry and geocoded prostate cancer mortality records from a state department of public health, we produce spatially continuous maps of indirectly age-adjusted late-stage prostate cancer and prostate cancer mortality maps of Iowa for the period 1999 through 2003. We show the sensitivity of these maps to differences in the four types of geocodes used to produce them.

For the prostate cancer late-stage maps, we compare maps produced with ZIP code-level geocoded data (940 areas) with maps produced from individual-level geocodes. For the prostate cancer mortality maps, we compare maps produced with county-level geocoded data (99 areas) with maps produced from city and rest of county geocoded data (1053 areas). The upscaling methods — used for the late-stage maps and one of the two types of mortality maps — employ fixed-distance filters and spatially adaptive filters (four parameters in all). The downscaling methods — used for one of the mortality maps — employ a commonly used spatial smoothing method. We discuss the usefulness of these maps in the context of cancer prevention and control activities. An appendix to the chapter describes the software we developed to make the computations on which the maps are based. The software is available from a publicly available Web site. These results are input to geographic information system (GIS) software to make the maps.

4.2 THE IMPORTANCE OF SPATIAL RESOLUTION
IN CANCER MAPS

There are a number of reasons for wanting cancer maps that are spatially continuous. Conceptually, we have no reasons to expect cancer rates to conform to the usually arbitrary areas for which data are mapped using commonly used choropleth mapping methods.[1] This means that anyone who uses a county-level cancer map should recognize that the cancer rates are undoubtedly spatially misaligned with respect to the true boundaries where changes in rates take place. We know this because the information has not been processed geographically by methods that could reveal the boundaries of change within the counties if they were there. Although this fact is known by many who make cancer maps,[2-4] removing the barriers that could remedy this fault has not received the attention it deserves. Two barriers are common: the lack of access to geocodes of the cancer data and related demographic data at a fine level of geographic resolution and the availability of GIS-based software to process the information and produce results of known levels of geographic accuracy and precision. This chapter shows that when custodians of cancer data — such as a cancer registry or a state department of public health — have such geocodes attached to their cancer records, they now have the means to see that cancer data are processed so that these geographic details are available wherever the data can support the methods described in this chapter.

The reason intracounty variability in cancer rates exists is that many risk factors for cancer are spatially variable within counties.[5,6] Likewise, many potential covariates of cancer risk are continuously distributed. Portraying cancer risk as spatially continuous also permits interpretation at multiple levels of spatial resolution so that exploration of spatial variations at different scales of analysis becomes possible. The methods for producing such maps depend, critically, on the availability of geocodes of different degrees of spatial resolution,[7] which permit makers of maps to use multiple scales of measurement, leading to maps at different spatial resolutions. The spatial variability of cancer rates occurs at multiple scales so that, during the course of an investigation, it may become necessary to change the scale at which rates are measured. We illustrate this point in this chapter.

This chapter explores multiple scales of measurement, the role of different geocodes, and the role of different methodologies and tools in producing these maps. It also correlates the maps produced by different geocodes and different methods for estimating rates and explores the conditions for which the resulting maps are similar or different. It is intuitively evident that geographic detail in a cancer map should relate to the unit size for which cancer data and population data are available. The relationship between scale of data and scale of the map, however, is complex. Two atlases of cancer, for example, show considerable geographic detail based on cancer data for large areas — counties in the case of Ohio and municipalities in the case of Finland.[8,9] The fine geographical detail shown in these atlases is achieved by spatial interpolation methods using kernel density estimation techniques that smooth the rates based on centroids of areas for which they have been calculated. The geographic detail of the map bears little resemblance to the geographic detail of the data; rather, it results from a model of the process of the (unknown) spatial variability of the cancer map. This method, commonly called *smoothing of rates*, has been described in detail previously.[10] Users of such maps often are uneasy when they see that the geographic detail on the map has been created by the model when the same geographic detail might have been measured more directly if cancer data had been available for smaller areas and if the process of spatial aggregation had been controlled. As Atkinson and Tate (p. 69) noted, "The commonly employed techniques of averaging, smoothing, extrapolation, and interpolating to different scales of measurement are hazardous."[11]

The validity of such maps depends on what is known about the process that generates them — the subject of much research in geographical analysis. The distinction is between the geographic detail produced by the spatial measurement method and the geographic detail produced by the model of spatial variation applied to calculated rates for predefined geographic regions (see reference 11). In both cases, there is a spatial basis of support for the rate observed at any point on the map, but the methodology for producing this rate is different. It would be nice to know the degree of error likely to be introduced by using the model to derive the spatial detail that measurement otherwise did not allow. Of course, there are circumstances when, often for purposes of privacy protection, the finest level of geographic detail cannot be

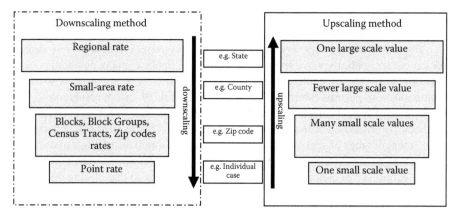

FIGURE 4.1 Alternative approaches for changing the spatial basis of support (COSP) in spatially continuous cancer maps

measured because this detail has been lost through the spatial aggregation process[12] (e.g., see reference 13). In this chapter, however, we explore the relative gain and loss through access to geocoded cancer data at different levels of spatial resolution. The aim is to produce results and to reach conclusions that will contribute to reducing the hazard incurred in using methods that attempt to reconstruct geographic detail after the original detail was lost in the spatial measurement process.

The reason for exploring spatial measurement issues is that the current literature has largely ignored them. As Gotway and Young noted, producing maps of disease inevitably involves a process of downscaling or upscaling spatial data.[7] This process is known as the change of support problem (COSP). Figure 4.1 illustrates that most cancer maps to date have been produced by a process of downscaling. In downscaling, rates are measured based on the support of large areas, and a model is used to produce rates for smaller areas than the support areas. The most common models used are spatial smoothing.[1,8–10,13] Unfortunately, these areas are frequently of different sizes, shapes, and populations, with the result that the fundamental measurement is made at different (variable) measurement scales, and a model is used to produce local geographical detail in the map. It is also common to note that the downscaling ought to adjust for variability in the measurement errors in the data used, although this adjustment is not always made, and there is not yet consensus on how it should be done. The purpose of any map is to provide an informative and accurate description of the spatial variation in cancer risk. Constructing maps on the basis of arbitrary and different measurement levels and geographic details produced by models of spatial variation that have little theoretical support are two undesirable characteristics of most current maps.

In upscaling, rates are based on point supports that become area-based supports based on geostatistical principles using area-to-point spatial interpolation methods.[14,15] The accuracy of the area-to-point predictions will depend on the loss of information incurred by the upscaling procedure involved in the spatial measurement model. All aggregations of the original observations result in loss of information because the spatial variation within the aggregation area is lost. This is a reason for keeping the geographic scale of the upscaling to a minimum. Evidence is provided here that particular combinations of geocode size and spatial filter definition can achieve this. In summary, there are four decisions to make when producing a spatially continuous cancer map:

- Select the type of rate to map.
- Select the geocode.
- Select the grid from which measurements of rates will be made.
- Select the spatial measurement method and key parameters — fixed distance or spatially adaptive.

The remainder of this chapter describes these choices and discusses the ways in which results are affected by them.

4.3 EFFECTS OF SPATIAL FILTER TYPE, SIZE, AND GEOCODE UNIT: LATE-STAGE PROSTATE CANCER RATES

In this section, we assess the validity and variability of cancer maps under different combinations of spatial filter types (fixed distance vs. adaptive) and geocode units (ZIP code vs. individual point). The spatial filter types are implemented in the software (DMAP IV) described in the appendix to this chapter.

Prostate cancer incidence data in Iowa (1998–2003) were used in this analysis. The data are from the Iowa Cancer Registry. For areas defined around regularly spaced grid points, we computed indirectly age-adjusted late-stage prostate cancer rates; the spatial filter method was described in 1996 by Rushton and Lolonis[16]; the indirect age-adjustment method, as used in a GIS context, was described in 1997 by Waller and McMaster.[17] That is, we computed late-stage rates for Iowa for 5-year male age groups (Table 4.1). We counted the total number of prostate cancer cases in the age

TABLE 4.1
Prostate Cancer Cases in Iowa by Age after Removing Unstaged Cases (1998–2003)

Age Groups	Prostate Cancer Cases	Late-Stage Percentage (%)
<50	193	6.2
50–54	643	10.4
55–59	1132	8
60–64	1734	7.6
65–69	2337	8.9
70–74	2510	8.7
75–79	2009	10.9
80–84	1137	15.7
85+	702	21.9
Overall	**12397**	**10.4**

TABLE 4.2
Combinations of Geographic Area,[a] Spatial Filter Types, and Geocoding Units for Prostate Cancer Late-Stage Maps

Combination	Geographic Area	Spatial Filter	Geocoding Level
1	Iowa	Adaptive (70 expected late-stage cases)	Individual cases
2	Iowa	Adaptive (70 expected late-stage cases)	Zip Code
3	Iowa	Fixed Distance (15 miles)	Individual cases
4	Iowa	Fixed Distance (15 miles)	Zip Code
5	Polk County	Adaptive (70 expected late-stage cases)	Individual cases
6	Polk County	Adaptive (70 expected late-stage cases)	Zip Code
7	Polk County	Fixed Distance (8 miles)	Individual cases
8	Polk County	Fixed Distance (8 miles)	Zip Code

[a] We used a 3-mile grid (6273 grid points) in computations for Iowa and a 1-mile grid (702 grid points) in computations for Polk County.

group in the filter area of each grid point and applied the statewide late-stage rate of this age group to this total to estimate the number of expected late-stage cases in the filter area in the age group. For each of the spatial filter areas, defined in several ways as specified in this chapter, we computed the ratio of observed late-stage cases to the expected number of late-stage cases, which is the standardized late-stage prostate cancer rate (SLR). A rate of 1.0 is interpreted to mean that the sum of the observed late-stage cases is equal to the sum of the expected late-stage cases in the defined filter area at the grid point in question. A rate larger than 1.0 indicates that the filter area had more late-stage incidences than would be expected using the statewide rate. In the maps reviewed, we computed the rate of late-stage prostate cancer for the grid points as defined in Table 4.2. We used SEER summary stage 1977 to define late-stage prostate cancer. Stage code 1 (localized) was classified as early stage, codes 5 (regional) and 7 (distant) were classified as late stage, code 9 (unstaged) records were excluded from the analysis (Table 4.3). We used four combinations of selected

TABLE 4.3
Prostate Cancer Cases in Iowa by Stage (1998–2003)

SEER Summary Stage 1977	Prostate Cancer Cases	Percentage
1	11117	85.13%
5	527	4.04%
7	763	5.76%
9	662	5.07%
Total	**13059**	**100%**

TABLE 4.4
Correlations of Estimated Late-Stage Prostate Proportions among Combinations 1–4

Iowa (6273 data points)	1. adap70_ind	2. adap70_zip	3. fix15_ind	4. fix15_zip
1. adap70_ind	1	N/A	N/A	N/A
2. adap70_zip	0.9783	1	N/A	N/A
3. fix15_ind	0.5458	0.5603	1	N/A
4. fix15_zip	0.5340	0.5459	0.9310	1

spatial filter types and geocoding levels to compute the indirectly age-adjusted late-stage prostate cancer proportions for two scales of geographical areas (Iowa and Polk County, where the state capital, Des Moines, is located) and so defined eight different cancer maps (Table 4.2). From computations at the grid points, the surface was interpolated using the inverse-distance-weighted (IDW) method in ArcGIS, using the six nearest neighbors of each grid point.

We used both summary statistics and maps to analyze the similarity and difference between the computed late-stage prostate cancer map estimates. We computed correlations among estimates from combinations 1, 2, 3, 4 and combinations 5, 6, 7, 8 separately to compare the overall similarity between different combinations of spatial filter and geocoding levels (Tables 4.4 and 4.5).

We computed the min, max, mean, and standard deviation measures of filter radius and the SLRs and their standard errors from the different combinations to compare their validity and variability (Tables 4.6 and 4.7).

TABLE 4.5
Correlations of Estimated Late-Stage Prostate Proportions among Combinations 5–8

Polk County (702 data points)	5. adap70_ind	6. adap70_zip	7. fix8_ind	8. fix8_zip
5. adap70_ind	1	N/A	N/A	N/A
6. adap70_zip	0.7598	1	N/A	N/A
7. fix8_ind	−0.0947	−0.0827	1	N/A
8. fix8_zip	−0.2146	−0.1514	0.8287	1

TABLE 4.6

Summary Statistics for the Filter Radius in the Spatial Adaptive Filter Approaches among Combinations 1, 2, 5, and 6

Combination	Variable	N	Min	Max	Mean	Std Dev
1. adap70_ind	Filter Radius (miles)	6273	4.9	77.1	37.53	10.73
2. adap70_zip	Filter Radius (miles)	6273	5.1	76.4	37.02	10.37
5. adap70_ind	Filter Radius (miles)	702	4.8	22.2	12.36	4.16
6. adap70_zip	Filter Radius (miles)	702	4.6	23.1	12.55	4.2

TABLE 4.7

Summary Statistics for the SLRs[a] and Their Standard Errors[b] from the Eight Combinations

Combination	Variable	N	Min	Max	Mean	Std Dev
1. adap70_ind	SLR[a]	6273	0.625	1.45	1.036	0.18
1. adap70_ind	SE(SLR)[b]	6273	0.094	0.143	0.121	0.009
2. adap70_zip	SLR	6273	0.617	1.53	1.039	0.185
2. adap70_zip	SE(SLR)	6273	0.088	0.148	0.121	0.012
3. fix15_ind	SLR	6273	0	2.936	1.061	0.357
3. fix15_ind	SE(SLR)	6273	0	1.186	0.321	0.126
4. fix15_zip	SLR	6273	0	2.848	1.058	0.37
4. fix15_zip	SE(SLR)	6273	0	1.255	0.323	0.134
5. adap70_ind	SLR	702	0.906	1.294	1.118	0.081
5. adap70_ind	SE(SLR)	702	0.116	0.139	0.129	0.004
6. adap70_zip	SLR	702	0.917	1.216	1.08	0.06
6. adap70_zip	SE(SLR)	702	0.113	0.133	0.124	0.004
7. fix8_ind	SLR	702	0	1.857	0.986	0.295
7. fix8_ind	SE(SLR)	702	0	0.758	0.256	0.143
8. fix8_zip	SLR	702	0	2.024	1.01	0.301
8. fix8_zip	SE(SLR)	702	0	0.85	0.265	0.165

[a] SLR refers to standardized late-stage prostate cancer rate.

[b] Equation for standard error of SLR is SE (SLR) = $\sqrt{\#\text{observed} / \#\text{expected}}$

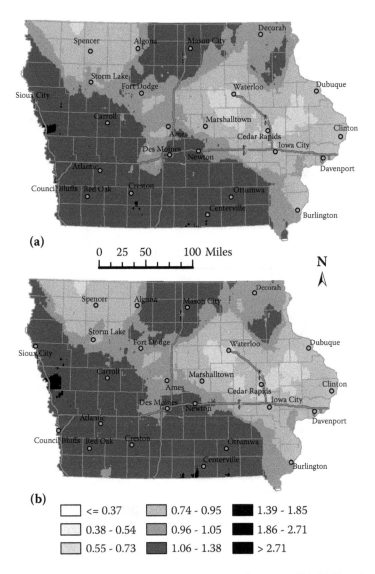

(a)

0   25   50   100 Miles

N

(b)

☐ <= 0.37	▦ 0.74 - 0.95	■ 1.39 - 1.85
☐ 0.38 - 0.54	▦ 0.96 - 1.05	■ 1.86 - 2.71
▦ 0.55 - 0.73	▦ 1.06 - 1.38	■ > 2.71

FIGURE 4.2 Standardized late-stage prostate cancer rate in Iowa (1998–2003) using adaptive filter of 70 expected late-stage cases: (a) individual case data (combination 1); (b) ZIP code-level data (combination 2).

We produced maps of the late-stage prostate cancer proportions and standard error maps for visual illustration and interpreted the results with summary statistics (see Figures 4.2–4.7). The number of observed and expected cases at all 6273 grid points do not equal the total cases observed because the spatial filter areas overlap and the same cases were counted many times. The benefit of this overlapping of

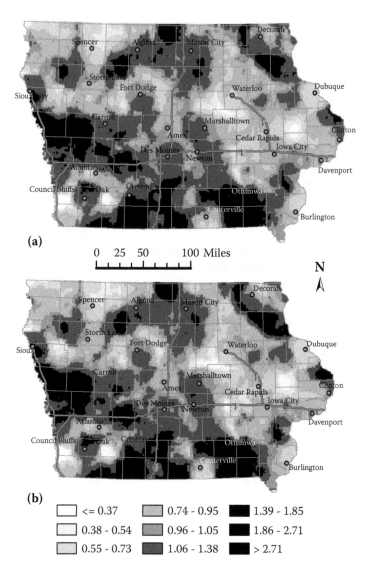

FIGURE 4.3 Standardized late-stage prostate cancer rate in Iowa (1998–2003) using a fixed-distance filter of 15 miles: (a) individual case data (combination 3); (b) ZIP code-level data (combination 4).

spatial measurement areas is that the method removes the zoning effect and controls the aggregation effect in the modifiable areal unit problem.[18] The method does not ensure, however, that the total number of observed cases will equal the total number of expected cases over the map. In Table 4.8, we show these totals over all grid points; filter areas are almost identical, and no significant bias was introduced by this process. The largest ratio of observed to expected is 1.04 for the largest spatially adaptive filter size of 70 late-stage individuals for both individual- and ZIP code-level geocoded data.

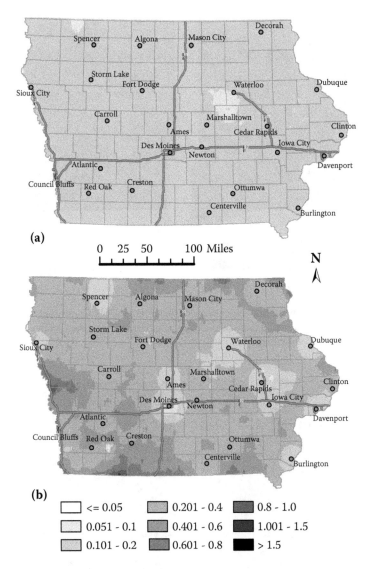

FIGURE 4.4 Standard error of the standardized late-stage prostate cancer rate in Iowa (1998–2003) using adaptive filter and fixed-distance filter: (a) adaptive filter (70 expected late-stage cases and individual data, combination 1); (b) fixed-distance filter (15 miles and individual data, combination 3).

4.3.1 RESULTS: ADAPTIVE SPATIAL FILTERS COMPARED WITH FIXED-DISTANCE SPATIAL FILTERS

The adaptive spatial filter method can stabilize the estimating error. The number of cases needed in a filter area to provide a given precision for the proportions can be estimated in advance. The expected number of 70 prostate late-stage incidences was computed as the minimum number required for the indirectly age-adjusted

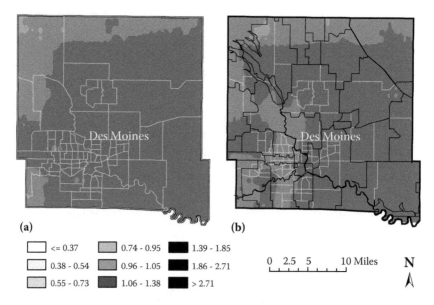

(a)   **(b)**

☐ <= 0.37	▨ 0.74 - 0.95	▰ 1.39 - 1.85
☐ 0.38 - 0.54	▨ 0.96 - 1.05	▰ 1.86 - 2.71
▨ 0.55 - 0.73	▨ 1.06 - 1.38	▰ > 2.71

0   2.5   5   10 Miles   N

FIGURE 4.5 Standardized late-stage prostate cancer rate in Polk County (1998–2003) using adaptive filter of 70 expected late-stage cases: (a) individual case data (combination 5); (b) ZIP code-level data (combination 6).

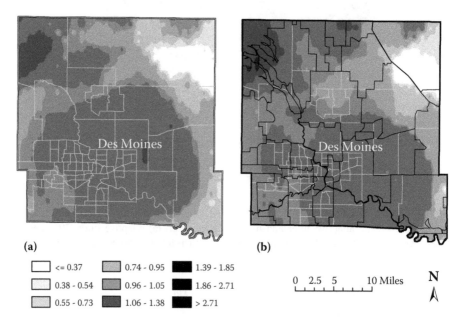

(a)   **(b)**

☐ <= 0.37	▨ 0.74 - 0.95	▰ 1.39 - 1.85
☐ 0.38 - 0.54	▨ 0.96 - 1.05	▰ 1.86 - 2.71
▨ 0.55 - 0.73	▨ 1.06 - 1.38	▰ > 2.71

0   2.5   5   10 Miles   N

FIGURE 4.6 Standardized late-stage prostate cancer rate in Polk County (1998–2003) using fixed-distance filter of 8 miles: (a) individual case data (combination 7); (b) ZIP code-level data (combination 8).

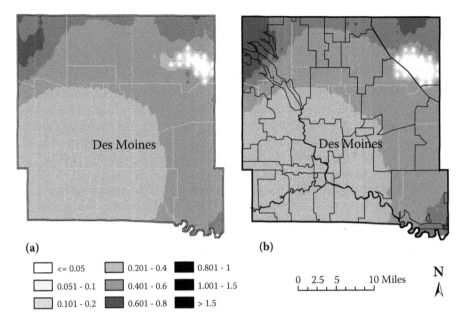

FIGURE 4.7 Standard error of the standardized late-stage prostate cancer rate in Polk County (1998–2003) using fixed-distance filter of 8 miles: (a) individual case data (combination 7); (b) ZIP code-level data (combination 8).

late-stage prostate cancer proportion to be within the 90% confidence interval of within plus or minus 0.2 times the estimated proportion value. The fixed distance spatial filters provide estimates of different degrees of precision, which is the principal disadvantage of this filter type (see Table 4.7 and Figure 4.4). We can also see that the spatial patterns of late-stage proportions change dramatically from fixed and adaptive filters (Tables 4.4 and 4.5; Figures 4.2, 4.3, 4.5, and 4.6). The filter

TABLE 4.8

Measuring Overall Bias from the Spatial Filter Methods: Difference between Total Observed Cases and Total Expected Cases among Combinations 1–4

Combination	Sum of Observed Late-Stage Cases Over All Grid Points	Sum Of Expected Late-Stage Cases Over All Grid Points	Total Observed/ Total Expected
1. adap70_ind	460020	442867.6	1.04
2. adap70_zip	456667	439971.2	1.04
3. fix15_ind	92099	91922	1.002
4. fix15_zip	91628	91643	0.999

size varies with data density in the adaptive spatial filter method (Table 4.6); the mean filter size is about 20–30 miles in this example.

4.3.2 GEOCODE SIZE: INDIVIDUAL DATA COMPARED WITH ZIP CODE DATA

From Figure 4.2 and Table 4.4, it is clear that, using the adaptive spatial filter, the late-stage cancer rates are remarkably similar whether the individual geocode or the ZIP code geocode is used. However, when the scale of the map is changed and the adaptive filter is applied to a smaller area of one county where population density is high, there are some noticeable differences between the maps (cf. Table 4.5 and Figure 4.5).

For the fixed-distance spatial filter, the results are similar at the state level when a relatively large (15-mile) filter size is used (Table 4.4, Figure 4.3). When a smaller (8-mile) filter is used, more difference in the computed SLRs and maps between those that use individual data and those using ZIP code data can be identified, such as a smaller correlation coefficient in Table 4.5 and more pattern difference in Figures 4.6 and 4.7.

4.3.3 CONCLUSIONS FOR THE LATE-STAGE MAPS

The adaptive spatial filter type is superior to the fixed-distance spatial filter type. Although it seems that we lose much spatial detail and see much less "extreme" SLR values (cf. Figures 4.2 and 4.3 and Table 4.7), we are more confident about our results. The effect of the geocoding level varies depending on the type of filter used and the size of the study area. The effect is minimal when a large adaptive filter is applied on a large area (Figure 4.2, Table 4.4), and the maximum is more evident when a small fixed-distance filter is applied on a smaller area (Figure 4.6, Table 4.5). Note that for all maps compared, an upscaling process was used. The change of spatial support is because of different relative sizes of the aggregated geocodes. Any point on the map is supported by a larger area than any of the geocodes. The rate values at any point are derived from data aggregated from smaller geocodes. Thus, the rate values portrayed are for overlapping spatial areas of data. This is the upscaling property that can be compared with the downscaling property in one of the prostate cancer mortality maps discussed in the next section.

4.4 EFFECTS OF SPATIAL FILTER TYPE, SIZE, AND GEOCODE UNIT: PROSTATE CANCER MORTALITY RATES

In this section, we assess the validity and variability of cancer maps under different combinations of spatial filter types (fixed distance vs. adaptive) and geocode units (counties vs. city codes and rest of county [rural areas]). This section is different from section 4.3 in that the source of the mortality data was the Iowa Department of Public Health, and the geocodes used are different from those used by the Iowa Cancer Registry. These differences permitted us to explore their effect on producing spatially continuous cancer maps. Disease-specific mortality data for Iowa are released for approved research projects following formal review by the Iowa Department of Public Health under a carefully supervised data-sharing agreement. Each case is assigned to two types of geographic references: the county, for which there are 99 in Iowa, and the city and "rest of county," for which there are a total of 1053 areas. Note that cancer deaths coded for the rural part of counties cover all areas of the county that are nonurban. Urban areas are legally defined, incorporated areas. These are unusual geocodes in that the rural component areas are spatially noncontiguous, and these are represented in this work by using the geometric centroid of each county. Deaths in the remaining areas of each county are represented by the coordinates of their respective urban area (city codes). To compute mortality rates for any area, however, it is necessary to ensure that the spatial alignment of the mortality data in the filter areas is exactly the same as the area from which the population data were assembled. When the mortality data originate with a state health department and the population data originate with the U.S. Census, there are possible problems with spatial misalignment between the geocodes even when they have the same names. It is not certain, for example, that persons completing a certificate of death, when stating place of residence of the death, conform in their naming of urban places to census definitions of urban areas.

4.4.1 RESULTS: ADAPTIVE SPATIAL FILTERS COMPARED WITH FIXED-DISTANCE SPATIAL FILTERS

Spatially continuous maps based on county-level geocodes can be produced only by a downscaling method. The size of the county-level geocodes precludes producing them by an upscaling process (see Figure 4.1). For each grid point on a 3-mile grid, we computed the indirect, age-adjusted mortality rate based on the data aggregated within the spatial filter area as variously defined (see Table 4.9). For the county geocodes, for each 5-year age-group, the mortality numbers were summed over all

TABLE 4.9
Combinations of Spatial Filter Types and Geocoding Units for Prostate Cancer Mortality Maps

Combination	Spatial Filter	Geocoding Level
1	Fixed Distance (30 miles)	99 counties
2	Fixed Distance (40 miles)	"
3	Adaptive (20 expected mortality cases)	"
4	Adaptive (37 expected mortality cases)	"
5	Fixed Distance (30 miles)	1053 combination of cities and rest of counties
6	Fixed Distance (40 miles)	"
7	Adaptive (20 expected mortality cases)	"
8	Adaptive (37 expected mortality cases)	"
9	Adaptive (60 expected mortality cases)	99 counties
10	Adaptive (60 expected mortality cases)	1053 combination of cities and rest of counties

counties with centroids that lay within the filter area, and for the same counties the population data (U.S. Census 2000) were summed. Expected numbers of deaths were computed using statewide, age-specific death rates (males only). To compute the values of map pixels between the grid points, as in section 4.3, we used the inverse-distance-weighted (IDW) smoothing method with eight nearest grid point neighbors as implemented in ArcGIS version 8.3. The results (Figure 4.8) show substantial differences in the spatial patterns of mortality between the map

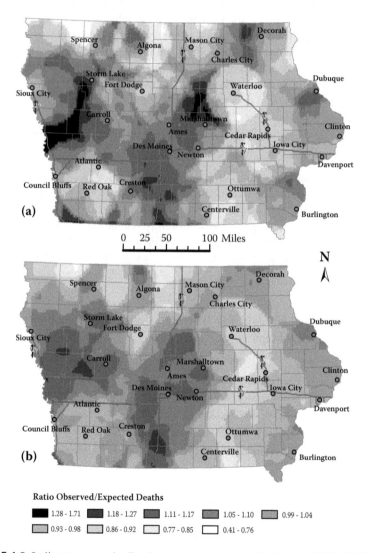

FIGURE 4.8 Indirect age standardized prostate cancer mortality in Iowa (1999–2003) using fixed-distance filters and county centroids for geocodes (99 areas; combinations 1 and 2): (a) 30-mile fixed-distance filter; (b) 40-mile fixed-distance filter.

TABLE 4.10

Correlation of Estimated Prostate Cancer
Mortality Rates between Combination 1 and 2

Pearson Correlation Coefficient, N = 6273
Prob > |r| under H0: Rho = 0

	Fix40_99
Fix30_99	0.6463(<.0001)

based on a 30-mile radius filter and one based on a 40-mile filter. Iowa counties are approximately 30 miles across, so that a 30-mile filter will generally pull in the centroids of all adjacent counties to any grid point, whereas the 40-mile filter will in some cases pull in more than the immediately adjacent counties. Consequently, Figure 4.8b is noticeably smoother than Figure 4.8a. The correlation between the 6300 grid point values for these two maps is 0.6463, indicating a substantial difference between the two map patterns (see Table 4.10).

4.4.2 GEOCODE SIZE: SMALL-AREA DATA COMPARED WITH COUNTY-LEVEL DATA

The geocodes for the areas smaller than counties are unusual in that records that carry the geocoded rest of county refer to all records not in the incorporated urban areas of the county. Records of persons who reside in the incorporated urban areas are geocoded to the centroid of each urban area. Because a U.S. Census tabulation of population data for counties is also available for rest-of-county designations, it is possible to compute mortality rates for all geocodes with centroids that fall within any filter area. When the centroid of a county is within a filter area, the mortality records and the population values for rest of county are assigned to the filter area and are aggregated together with the data for other urban areas in the area before computing the mortality rate for the area. When these geocodes are used, the correlation (r = .7308) between the 30-mile and 40-mile filter area maps increased, indicating that a substantial part of the difference in patterns between the maps was caused by the grossness of the county-level geocodes (see Figure 4.9). As with the county-level geocodes, the 40-mile filter area map is noticeably smoother than the 30-mile area map.

The four mortality maps in Figures 4.10 and 4.11 were all constructed using spatially adaptive filters. In Figure 4.10, the comparison is between the county-level geocodes (Figure 4.10a) and the more disaggregated geocodes (Figure 4.10b). The adaptive filters meet the criterion of a minimum of 60 expected deaths. The more detailed spatial definition of Figure 4.10b illustrates the gain by use of the small spatial resolution of the geocodes compared with county geocodes in Figure 4.10a. Figures 4.10b, 4.11a, and 4.11b merit comparison because they are all based on the smaller spatial data geocodes and differ only from the use of different threshold numbers for expected deaths in the spatial filters. Increased smoothing is apparent in the order of Figure 4.11a to 4.11b to 4.10b.

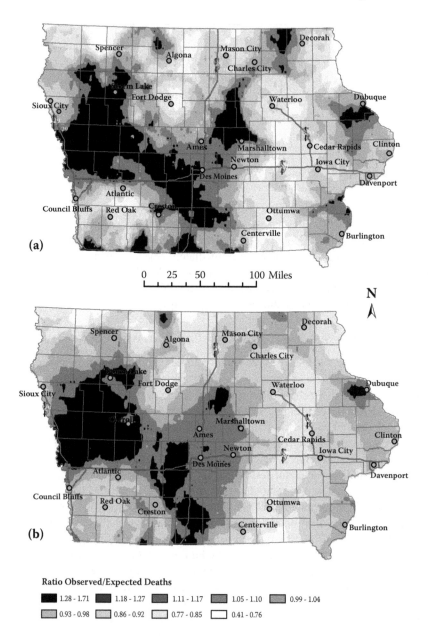

FIGURE 4.9 Indirect age-standardized prostate cancer mortality in Iowa (1999–2003) using fixed-distance filters and city and rural geocodes (1053 areas; combinations 5 and 6): (a) 30-mile fixed-distance filter; (b) 40-mile fixed-distance filter.

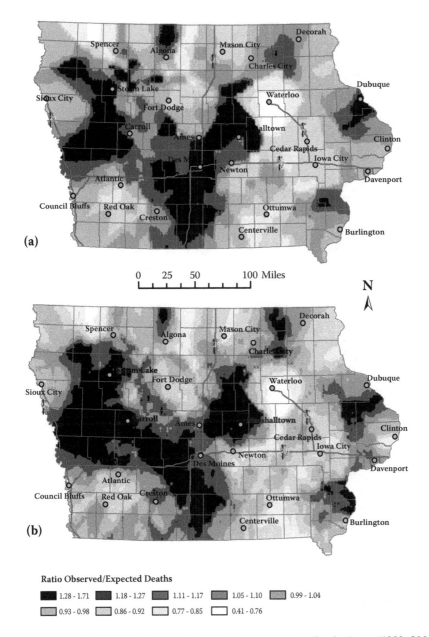

FIGURE 4.10 Indirect age-standardized prostate cancer mortality in Iowa (1999–2003) using adaptive filters and county versus city and rural geocodes (combinations 9 and 10): (a) adaptive filters of 60 expected deaths with county geocodes; (b) adaptive filters of 60 expected deaths with city and rural geocodes.

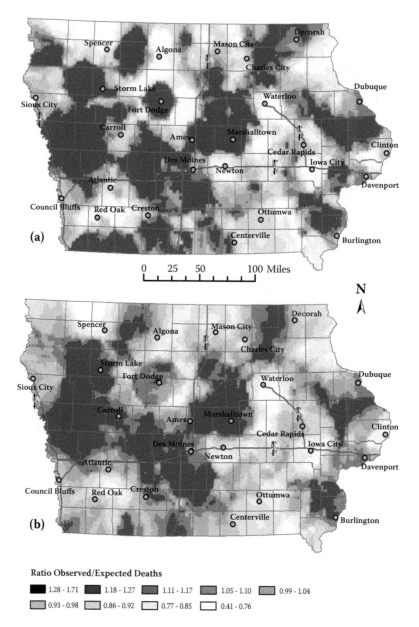

FIGURE 4.11 Indirect age-standardized prostate cancer mortality in Iowa (1999–2003) using adaptive filters and city and rural geocodes (1053 areas; combinations 7 and 8): (a) adaptive filters of 20 expected deaths; (b) adaptive filters of 37 expected deaths.

4.4.3 CONCLUSIONS FOR THE PROSTATE CANCER MORTALITY MAPS

The prostate mortality map series shows that spatial detail in the maps is gained by the process of disaggregation in the size of the spatial units for mortality and population even when one of the spatial units describing the nonurban population continues to be coded at a coarser spatial resolution than the urban population component.

4.5 CONCLUSIONS: REMOVING THE BARRIERS TO PRODUCING SPATIALLY CONTINUOUS CANCER MAPS

In this chapter, we have demonstrated that it is possible to produce cancer maps with better geographic resolution and known accuracy of rates using geocoded cancer data at fine degrees of geographic resolution. We showed that for all areas except large urban areas, ZIP code geocodes provided geographic resolutions for late-stage maps that were almost indistinguishable from the geographic resolution of maps produced from individual geocoded cancer records. Although this conclusion may not be generalized to all areas, it surely supports a finding that such maps can be produced from cancer data at some degree of spatial aggregation. Because most cancer maps also require the spatial alignment of demographic data with the cancer data, and demographic data are only available for selected geographic units, this result is important in practice. We also showed that numbers of expected cancer cases, known to provide a given level of accuracy of cancer rates, can be used to define optimal spatial filters — called spatially adaptive filters — to make the spatially continuous maps. We conclude that the barriers to producing spatially continuous cancer maps with valid geographical detail, discussed in section 4.1, can be removed.

The problem for the user of continuous cancer maps is that the geographical detail shown on the map does not necessarily correspond to the geographical detail that exists. The map by itself does not provide the information to judge its usefulness. In particular, when the geographical detail is produced by downscaling from large geocoded data units such as counties, the geographical detail shown is often far more than is warranted from the geographical resolution of the cancer data that supported its production. "Caveat emptor" should be prominently placed on such maps. We conclude that the future of cancer mapping lies in methods of spatial data analysis that control the spatial basis of support for all rates displayed by employing geographic measurement models based on individual-level or small-area-level geocoded cancer data and carefully selected parameters for the spatially adaptive filters on which they are based. The significance of this conclusion is that these improved cancer maps can be used in cancer prevention and control activities. Abed et al. (2000) described a framework for making decisions in this area, most of which are about what to do and where to do it.[19] These maps provide the best decision support device currently known for making these key location decisions.

REFERENCES

1. Devesa, S. S.; Grauman, D. J.; Blot, W. J.; Pennello, G.; Hoover, R. N.; Fraumeni, J. F., Jr. *Atlas of Cancer Mortality in the United States, 1950–94* [NIH Publication No. (NIH) 99-4564]. U.S. Government Printing Office, Washington, DC, 1999.
2. Bell, B. S.; Hoskins, R. E.; Pickle, L. W.; Wartenberg, D. Current practices in spatial analysis of cancer data: mapping health statistics to inform policymakers and the public. *International Journal of Health Geographics,* 5, 49, 2006.
3. Goovaerts, P. Geostatistical analysis of disease data: estimation of cancer mortality risk from empirical frequencies using Poisson kriging. *International Journal of Health Geographics,* 4, 31, 2005.
4. Lawson, A. B.; Biggeri, A. B.; Boehning, D.; Lesaffre, E.; Viel, J. F.; Clark, A.; Schlattmann, P.; Divino, F. Disease mapping models: an empirical evaluation. Disease Mapping Collaborative Group. *Statistics in Medicine,* 19, 2217–2241, 2000.
5. Berke, O. Exploratory disease mapping: kriging the spatial risk function from empirical Bayesian estimates of regional counts. *International Journal of Health Geographics,* 3, 18, 2004.
6. Goovaerts, P. Geostatistical analysis of disease data: accounting for spatial support and population density in the isopleth mapping of cancer mortality risk using area-to-point Poisson kriging. *International Journal of Health Geographics,* 5, 52, 2006.
7. Gotway, C. A.; Young, L. J. Combining incompatible spatial data. *Journal of the American Statistical Association,* 97, 632–648, 2002.
8. Pukkala, E.; Gustavsson, N.; Teppo, L. *Atlas of Cancer Incidence in Finland 1953–1982*. Cancer Society of Finland, Helsinki, 1987, Vol. 37.
9. Tyczynski, J. E.; Pasanen, K.; Berkel, H. J.; Pukkala, E. *Atlas of Cancer in Ohio: Incidence and Mortality*. Cancer Prevention Institute, Columbus, OH, 2006.
10. Kafadar, K. Smoothing geographical data, particularly rates of disease. *Statistics in Medicine,* 15, 2539–2560, 1996.
11. Atkinson, P. M.; Tate, N. J. Spatial scale problems and geostatistical solutions: a review. *Professional Geographer,* 52, 607–623, 2000.
12. Boscoe, F. P.; Ward, M. H.; Reynolds, P. Current practices in spatial analysis of cancer data: data characteristics and data sources for geographic studies of cancer. *International Journal of Health Geographics,* 3, 28, 2004.
13. Müller, H.-G.; Stadtmüller, U.; Tabnak, F. Spatial smoothing of geographically aggregated data, with application to the construction of incidence maps. *Journal of the American Statistical Association,* 92, 61–71, 1997.
14. Kyriakidis, P. C. A geostatistical framework for area-to-point spatial interpolation. *Geographical Analysis,* 36, 259–289, 2004.
15. Kyriakidis, P. C.; Yoo, E. H. Geostatistical prediction and simulation of point values from areal data. *Geographical Analysis,* 37, 124–151, 2005.
16. Rushton, G.; Lolonis, P. Exploratory spatial analysis of birth defect rates in an urban population. *Statistics in Medicine,* 15, 717–726, 1996.
17. Waller, L. A.; McMaster, R. B. Incorporating indirect standardization in tests for disease clustering in a GIS environment. *Geographical Systems,* 4, 327–342, 1997.
18. Wang, D. W. S. Aggregation effects in geo-referenced data. In *Advanced Spatial Statistics*, Griffith, D. A., Ed. CRC Press, Boca Raton, FL, 1996, pp. 83–106.
19. Abed, J.; Reilley, B.; Butler, M. O.; Kean, T.; Wong, F.; Hohman, K. Developing a framework for comprehensive cancer prevention and control in the United States: an initiative of the Centers for Disease Control and Prevention. *Journal of Public Health Management Practice,* 6, 67–78, 2000.

Appendix: DMAP IV — Software for Producing Disease Rates for Grid Points Based on Fixed Size or Adaptive Spatial Filters

Qiang Cai

PURPOSE

The DMAP IV (Disease Mapping and Analysis Program, Version IV) software is used to make kernel density estimates for spatial filters with either fixed geographical size or variable geographical size (adaptive). In the adaptive filter, the user selects the geographical size filter that contains a fixed number of cases (for geocoded point data) or that contains a minimum number of cases (for geocoded aggregate data). An example of aggregated data is ZIP codes for which ZIP code centroids are specified. Input can be data for points or aggregates of areas for which centroids are provided.

METHODOLOGY

The method (fixed spatial filter part) was originally developed in 1996 by Rushton and Lolonis.[1] This software also implements the adaptive spatial filter method.[2] The procedure can be summarized in the following four steps.

1. Define a set of grid points for the study area.
2. Draw fixed (or adaptive) distance circles around each grid point and count the number of cases (numerator: late-stage cancers) and population at risk (denominator: all cases of the cancer) for the study period. Of course, any data may be specified respectively as numerator and denominator data.
3. Compute rates at each grid point using results from step 2 (cases divided by population at risk; that is, numerator totals divided by denominator totals). To avoid the small-number problem, rates are not computed for grid points with insufficient at-risk population (by empirical judgment) within their supports. This value is an input parameter. The program

computes the rates at each grid point for which the denominator total exceeds the minimum input value. A contour or surface map is produced by spatially interpolating the rates at the grid points using a GIS.

4. Assume each individual within the population at risk has equal chance of being a case event. Use Monte Carlo simulation to compute a reference distribution of rates at each grid point, and an empirical p value of the observed rate is computed by comparing the observed rate with the reference distribution at this grid point. That is, at each grid point, the program computes the percentage of the simulated rates that are less than the observed rate value. This output can be mapped as a contour map by spatially interpolating the rates at the grid points using a GIS.

SPECIFICATIONS

The program needs two data files as inputs:

1. *Spatial Grid File:* Includes three fixed data fields: Grid ID, Longitude, Latitude.

2a. *Single-Point File:* Includes four fixed data fields (*Point ID, Longitude, Latitude, Disease* [0/1 value]) and some extra data fields, like *disease probability.*

OR

2b. *Spatial Centroid File:* If the original observations are not single spatial points, then the program needs a *Spatial Centroid File* instead of a *Single-Point File.* The *Spatial Centroid File* includes five fixed data fields (*Centroid ID, Longitude, Latitude, Disease counts, non-Disease counts*) and some extra data fields, like *Expected Disease counts.*

When the source data are individual data, data file 2a is used in the computation instead of data file 2b.

The data file format needs to be either a comma-delimitated text document (.txt) or a comma-separated values (.csv) file.

The program computes a rate file with the format of comma-separated values (.csv); this output includes seven fixed data fields (*Grid ID, Longitude, Latitude, Numerator, Denominator, Rate, Filter_radius*) and some more fields like *p-value* and *95% CIs,* depending on whether the user chooses to perform a Monte Carlo simulation.

EXAMPLE OF SOFTWARE INTERFACE

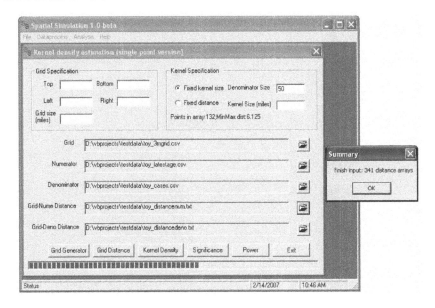

REFERENCES

1. Rushton, G.; Lolonis, P. Exploratory spatial analysis of birth defect rates in an urban population. *Statistics in Medicine*, 15, 717–726, 1996.
2. Talbot, T. O., Kulldorff, M., Forand, S. P., Haley, V. B. Evaluation of spatial filters to create smoothed maps of health data. *Statistics in Medicine,* 19, 2399–2408, 2000.

5 The Science and Art of Geocoding

Tips for Improving Match Rates and Handling Unmatched Cases in Analysis

Francis P. Boscoe

CONTENTS

5.1   INTRODUCTION

Given the breadth and detail of databases, maps, and other reference materials in existence, it is nearly always possible to find the physical location where a cancer patient resides. This task becomes easier with each passing year as the quality of hospital data improves, as address reference files improve, and as rural route and post office box addresses are gradually phased out to facilitate emergency response. Geo-codes can now be automatically assigned to well over 90% of incoming case reports in certain urban and suburban areas. For the remaining records, a modest amount of detective work is often all that is required to assign a geocode. But, when a large num-ber of records are involved, even a modest amount of detective work per case translates into an enormous amount of manual labor. Central cancer registries do not necessarily have the resources for such an effort, and there are always more pressing data quality concerns than precisely locating the most elusive fraction of the population.

A certain amount of missing geographic information is thus unavoidable. In this chapter, I discuss some non-labor-intensive ways to minimize missing geographic information. I then discuss some commonsense ways of incorporating ungeocoded records into epidemiological analyses. My examples are drawn primarily from New York State. Admittedly, New York is a comparatively easy state for geocoding — rural route addresses have been eliminated, and addresses with only a post office box are becoming gradually less common as municipalities that do not offer home mail delivery are increasingly urging residents to include both their post office box and their street name and number on their mail. Also, the New York State Department of Transportation, in conjunction with various public and private partners, recently completed a high-quality street coverage of the state that has resulted in substantially improved geocoding match rates. Still, there remain rural corners of the state where geocoding continues to present a significant challenge. As such, the points made in this chapter should be of value to central cancer registries even in primarily rural states.

5.2   MINIMIZING THE NUMBER OF UNGEOCODED RECORDS

There are a number of steps a cancer registry can take to minimize the number of ungeocoded records. These include the visual inspection of ungeocoded records to identify systematic problems, address standardization, refining matching algo-rithms, empirical geocoding, and detailed clerical review.

5.2.1   VISUAL INSPECTION OF UNGEOCODED RECORDS

Several years ago, my colleagues and I conducted an experiment to find out just why roughly one-fifth of the incoming address records sent to the New York State Cancer Registry were not automatically geocoded.[1] Before carrying out the experiment, we assumed that the most common reasons would be addresses with rural routes or post office boxes and the use of institutional or corporate names like Maple Hills Retire-ment Center or Van Dyck Apartments. Although our sample contained examples of each of these, we were surprised to learn that overwhelmingly the most common single reason (50% of the ungeocoded records in our sample) were addresses that were entirely correct but missing from our commercially obtained reference file. About one-fifth of these proved to be recently built homes on recently built streets, which presumably would have eventually geocoded with a future release of the ref-erence file. A majority, however, were addresses that had been around for decades, in both urban and rural areas. An entire small street in the South Bronx was absent; another street in Brooklyn had its last four blocks truncated.

The reasons for this had to do with uneven improvements in the reference file over time. The file had its ultimate origin in the coarse and error-laden 1990 street files published by the Census Bureau, with subsequent improvements driven largely by the needs of retailers and market researchers. This meant that mistakes and omissions in marginal economic areas were less likely to be corrected. We discovered this pattern by simply sorting the list of addresses that did not geocode by ZIP code and street name and noting groups of similar addresses that appeared to have nothing wrong with them. A call to our vendor verified our hypothesis.

Visual inspection of ungeocoded records led to the identification of other problems as well, including a number of commonly used abbreviations and punctuation quirks that were flummoxing our geocoding software. In many neighborhoods in Queens, New York City, hyphens are commonly used in house numbers, such as 113-78 120th Street. Standardizing the addresses to remove the hyphen solved the problem and revealed a smaller number of addresses with a space in place of the hyphen, such as 113 78 120th Street. The many "beach" addresses in the Rockaway Peninsula section of Queens (of the form 123 Beach 78th Street) were also not geocoded in the many instances when Beach was abbreviated BCH. Along Manhattan's fashionable Fifth Avenue, few people's addresses were geocoded because of a problem related to differing ZIP codes on opposite sides of the street (the problem was not unique to Fifth Avenue, but more cases were affected here than on any other street in the state). Each time I have thought that we had surely identified all possible systematic geocoding problems, I have been proven wrong. Thus, as long as there continue to be ungeocoded records, it is worth periodically reviewing them as a group to see if there are any unusual patterns.

5.2.2 ADDRESS STANDARDIZATION

Address standardization refers to the process of modifying an address so that it conforms to conventions for format, abbreviation, and address components. These conventions are defined by the U.S. Postal Service (USPS) in Publication 28.[2] Figure 5.1 shows a hypothetical address with the maximum possible number of address components. (North Canton, Ohio, is one of the few places in the country where streets may have both predirectionals and postdirectionals). Publication 28 also includes standards for addresses with post office boxes, rural routes, and other specialized situations. A central cancer registry record conforming to North American Association

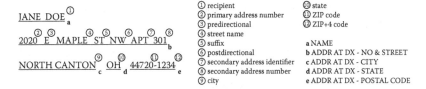

FIGURE 5.1 Standard address components (numbered) and NAACCR fields (lettered). Note that there are also corresponding NAACCR fields for current address, which may be different from the address at diagnosis.

of Central Cancer Registries (NAACCR) standards for cancer registries would store the address information in five fields, also indicated in the figure.[3]

A large variety of software exists that is able to take address information, parse it into its different address components, and modify these components to conform to the standard abbreviations listed in Publication 28 as well as make minor spelling corrections. This functionality is a standard feature of commercial geocoding software products, and there are also stand-alone software products entirely dedicated to address standardization. One benchmark of the quality of address standardizing software is whether it has been certified by the USPS Coding Accuracy Support System (CASS). Software that has been CASS certified has successfully matched 98% or more records in a standard test data set that is representative of all of the different address types in the country. Documentation on CASS is available at http://ribbs.usps.gov/files/cass/casstech.pdf.

Regardless of how a registry is standardizing its addresses, it is important to have the ability to make customized rules to reflect specific local situations. For example, in New York we have customized our software to standardize BWAY as Broadway, BX as Bronx when it appears in the city field, and MLK as Martin Luther King.

5.2.3 Refining Matching Algorithms

Another way of improving match rates is to refine the matching algorithms employed. Matching may be either *deterministic* or *probabilistic*. With the deterministic approach, one or more of the address components in the unmatched address are compared with the same address components in the reference file, and they must agree exactly and uniquely for a match to be made. With probabilistic matching, multiple address components are compared, with each component having a different weight. The weights for the components that match are then summed to obtain an overall match score, which is sometimes represented as a standardized number ranging from 0 (no elements match) to 100 (all elements match). These methods form part of a broader set of statistical methods known as record linkage and are not unique to geocoding or to public health. For further details of these methods, an excellent starting point is Howard B. Newcombe's *Handbook of Record Linkage*.[4]

The easiest way to illustrate the difference between these two methods is through an example. I use 1060 West Addison Street in Chicago, which is the address of Wrigley Field, a professional baseball stadium.

5.2.3.1 Deterministic Matching

A deterministic match typically consists of several passes, each with slightly more relaxed matching requirements:

> *Pass 1: Match on house number, predirectional, street name, suffix, ZIP code, and county.* In this first pass, only the exact string 1060 W Addison St, Chicago 60613 (Cook County) would geocode.
> *Pass 2: Match on house number, predirectional, street soundex, suffix, ZIP code, and county.* The soundex function is a way of representing a word based on its first letter and primary consonants, so that, in general, similar-sounding

words have the same code.[4] In this pass, 1060 W Attison St would geocode because it has the same soundex as Addison. However, if there were otherwise identical addresses in the same ZIP code with the same soundex, such as both 1060 W Addison St and 1060 W Atkinson St, then no unique match would result.

Pass 3: Same as pass 1, minus suffix. Here, 1060 W Addison, 1060 W Addison Ave, or 1060 W Addison Dr would geocode.

Pass 4: Same as pass 1, minus predirectional. In this instance, 1060 Addison St would geocode as long as there was not also a 1060 E Addison St in the same ZIP code, in which case the match would not be unique.

Pass 5: Same as pass 1, but replace ZIP code with City Name. Here, 1060 W Addison St Chicago 60614 (or any other ZIP code) would geocode. ZIP code errors in cities with multiple ZIP codes are fairly common; 13 of the 500 records in the New York State Cancer Registry geocoding study had this specific problem. Intriguingly, these errors tend to be from the nearest adjacent ZIP code rather than a random ZIP code in the city, suggesting the error is the result of an incorrect guess rather than a typographical error.

There are many more possible passes that could be made that would yield additional matches, but as the matching criteria become more relaxed, there is a larger chance of making an incorrect match. Pass 3 carries a small risk of error, for example, in cities where street names are repeated, which is a common legacy of cities' annexation of adjacent suburbs. In Pittsburgh, Pennsylvania, Main Street and North/South Main Street are 5 miles apart; both were the Main Streets of their respective boroughs before annexation to the city. Usually when street names are repeated, the house number ranges do not overlap, but there are exceptions. In Albany, New York, 101 3rd Avenue and 101 3rd Street are nowhere near each other, much to the bane of the occasional taxi driver or, more problematically, the occasional ambulance.

Albany's 3rd Avenue is in ZIP code 12202, and 3rd Street is in ZIP code 12210. A patient record listing 3rd Avenue 12210 could have either the suffix or the ZIP code incorrect. I have reviewed a number of these types of records and have found that either error is about equally likely. Based on pass 3, 3rd Avenue 12210 would be matched to 3rd Street 12210; based on pass 5, it would match to 3rd Avenue 12202. Because pass 3 precedes pass 5, the former match would prevail. The costs of making an error of this type must be weighed against the benefits of the number of correct geocodes that result from each step.

5.2.3.2 Probabilistic Matching

The probabilistic matching method requires the assignment of a weight to each field compared. The weight is derived from two probabilities. The first is the probability that two fields agree given that they are truly a match, denoted as m. In general, this probability will be high, close to 1. For example, if the true street name is Maple, then we would expect the majority of all associated patient records also to have the name Maple, but there may be a few with Mapple or some other minor spelling variation. The second probability is the probability that two fields agree at random, denoted as u. This probability is typically low. The New York State street file that

I currently work with has about 1.2 million street segments, of which about 3500 have the name Maple. Thus, the probability of a randomly selected record having the name Maple given one record with this name is about .003. In many states, there are only four permissible values in the predirectional field (N, S, E, W), making this *u* probability ¼.

Once *m* and *u* are known, the weight for each field can be calculated as

$$\text{Weight} = \ln (m/u)$$

Thus, for street name, assuming an *m* of .98 and a *u* of .003, the weight would be 5.79. For predirectional, using an *m* of .99 and a *u* of .25, the weight would be 1.38. Intuitively, it makes sense that the street name should be weighted much more heavily than the predirectional.

By way of example, suppose we wish to match on house number (assume a weight of 6.9), predirectional (1.4), street name (5.5), street soundex (5.1), suffix (1.5), ZIP code (6.2), and county (3.4). The address 1060 W Addison St 60613 (Cook County) would have the maximum match score of 30 because all elements match. The address 1060 W Attison St 60613 (Cook County) would have a score of 24.5 for differing only in the name field; 1060 W Addison St 60614 (Cook County) would score 23.8 for having the wrong ZIP code. Note that the score of interest is the *maximum* of all the candidate matches. Each of the examples has a score at least 3.4 when matched against every single address in Cook County and 9.6 when matched against every single address in the 60613 ZIP code, but these are of no interest.

Because this method calculates a match score for every address in the reference file, it is computationally intensive. A strategy known as *blocking* is used to eliminate the majority of candidate matches from consideration to speed up the process. Blocked variables must agree for a comparison to be made. Supposing that street soundex is used as the blocking variable, then Addison would only be compared with the set of streets with the same soundex. In the case of the New York street file, this would mean reducing the number of required match score calculations from 1.2 million to a mere 100. This step may seem too limiting (suppose the case record is 1060 W Madison or 1060 W Radison), but it is only the first step. Subsequent passes blocking on fields such as county or ZIP code could then be attempted on the remaining records.

All geocoding software employs some combination of the above methods or similar variants. It is important for central cancer registries to understand how the process works and whether it might be improved. Whether a deterministic or probabilistic approach is better depends on the particular data sets involved, although one study found that the probabilistic approach determines more correct matches but at the expense of incorrectly identifying some nonmatches as matches.[5] In geocoding terms, this means that probabilistic matching will geocode more records, mostly correctly but occasionally incorrectly.

5.2.4 Empirical Geocoding

Empirical geocoding refers to the practice of using already-geocoded records as a basis for geocoding additional records. In other words, the cancer registry itself is made to function as a geocoding reference file. This is particularly useful when encountering institutional names used in address fields. For example, suppose an incoming address record reads Shady Grove Nursing Home. Because this is not a postally acceptable address, lacking both a number and street, it will not be automatically geocoded. Eventually, someone on the cancer registry staff notices this and corrects it by looking up and entering the proper street address for the facility, moving Shady Grove Nursing Home to the supplemental address field.

Now imagine that over the course of the year eight more case records are received with the identical address of Shady Grove Nursing Home. If the contents of the registry address and supplemental address fields are scanned as part of the geocoding process, then a match will be found based on the original manually corrected record. Note that this process must take the ZIP code into account because institutional names are often repeated within a state. In addition to helping geocode residents of nursing homes and retirement facilities, this technique is useful for geocoding residents of public housing complexes, trailer parks, and campgrounds. It is also useful for informal or unofficial street names or streets with more than one official name, such as County Route 29 and River Road.

5.2.5 DETAILED CLERICAL REVIEW

A final strategy for resolving unmatched records is simply to review each of the records individually. This is labor intensive and may not be a realistic solution for every cancer registry. It is a critical step, though, when conducting a focused local study for which high precision and accuracy are essential, such as a study of cases residing within a fixed distance of a hazardous site. This approach can yield extremely high match rates. In the previously cited New York study,[1] we were able to locate census tracts for all but 1 case in a 500-case sample, with 32 of these identified through labor-intensive methods. (Few of these cases had post office boxes or rural route addresses; I more recently repeated the exercise in a single rural county and was able to locate census tracts for 93 of 111 ungeocoded cases.) More impressively, McElroy et al.[6] used online people-finding sites and mapping engines to assign latitude and longitude coordinates to 20% of a sample of 14,804 breast cancer patients in Wisconsin, resulting in an overall match rate of 97%.

Resources available for tracking down individual addresses include online telephone directories and people-finding Web sites. These continue to evolve rapidly so that any attempt to list examples here would be doomed to obsolescence. Many central cancer registries have access to their state's Department of Motor Vehicles database, typically on a one-at-a-time lookup basis. Other useful resources cited in canvassing of central registries included voter lists, death certificates, property tax records, state police records, and Alaska Permanent Fund Dividend applications.

5.3 HANDLING UNMATCHED RECORDS IN ANALYSIS

Inevitably, even with the best possible reference databases and best matching algorithms, there will always remain some unmatched records. Researchers have typically handled these unmatched records in two ways: excluding them from the analysis or placing them at the centroid of the smallest geographic area for which there is information, typically the ZIP code. (In New York State, over 99.99% of incoming case reports include a ZIP code, with other state registries reporting comparable numbers.) A third and less-commonly used option is to assign a location making use of known information about age, race, and ethnicity. This assigned location can either be an area, such as a census tract or census block group, or a point location. Each of these solutions has certain advantages and limitations.

5.3.1   EXCLUDING UNMATCHED RECORDS

Exclusion of unmatched records is by far the simplest solution — if a record cannot be geocoded, then delete it from the study. Studies taking this approach sometimes justify this action on the grounds that the number of deleted cases is relatively small (often in the 10%–20% range), and that the deleted cases have similar characteristics as the retained cases in terms of age, sex, race/ethnicity, stage at diagnosis, or other variables. Most often, no explicit justification is given. But for analyses spanning large geographical areas, there is one major difference between the included and excluded cases — the excluded cases will be disproportionately located in rural areas. Rural areas contain all of the ungeocodable rural route addresses, along with the bulk of post office box addresses, unofficial or informal street names, and streets absent from commercial reference files. Even in states such as New York that have replaced rural routes with standard addresses as part of an effort to improve the delivery of emergency services to rural areas, this remains true, as seen in Table 5.1.

Excluding over one-third of the cases in a study, as would be the case in the 10 least-populous counties of New York State, carries a great risk of selection bias. In the least-populous counties of New York, the 64.7% of cases that are geocoded are largely in compact towns and villages; the 35.3% that are ungeocoded largely reside in the surrounding countryside. Between town and countryside, there are differences in the age structure of the population, socioeconomic status, distance to treatment, and occupational and environmental exposures that could bias analytical results. Geographic selection bias is something best avoided if possible. When it cannot be avoided, it may be possible to reduce its effects on analytical results; see chapter 10 of this volume for details.

TABLE 5.1

Percentage of Cases Geocoded in New York State Cancer Registry, Diagnosis Year 2001, as of December 2004

Geographic Area	% Geocoded
10 most populous counties	91.8
10 least populous counties	64.7
Statewide	88.1

5.3.2 ASSIGN THE CENTROID OF THE SMALLEST GEOGRAPHIC UNIT AVAILABLE

A *geographic centroid* is a point location that represents the average location of a geographic area. Typically, in commercial geographic information system (GIS) software packages, it is defined as the point halfway between the northern and southern extents and halfway between the eastern and western extents of an area. This can vary depending on how the shape of the area is generalized and whether uninhabited parts of the area such as water and parkland are included. Various boundary files for Manhattan place the centroid at various locations in Central Park, spanning nearly a mile, including one in the south wing of the Metropolitan Museum of Art. So, although centroids are often taken to be precise, this is not actually the case, and they may fall in locations that are atypical of the geographic area as a whole. A geographic centroid can even fall outside its geographic area, as is true for the state of Florida, where the centroid lies well into the Gulf of Mexico. In such instances, GIS software typically will relocate the centroid to the nearest point within the geographic area (e.g., the nearest point on the Gulf shoreline).

A *population-weighted centroid* is a point representing the average location of all of the people in an area and is of greater utility in cancer surveillance and research, although it may differ little from the geographic centroid in areas of moderate to high population density. Because the locations of individual people are typically unavailable, population-weighted centroids are calculated by using the smallest available geographic unit, usually the census block. In ZIP code 12180, which includes most of the city of Troy, New York, as well as parts of several surrounding towns, the locations of the population-weighted centroid and the geographic centroid are far apart (Figure 5.2). The population-weighted centroids of subgroups within the population

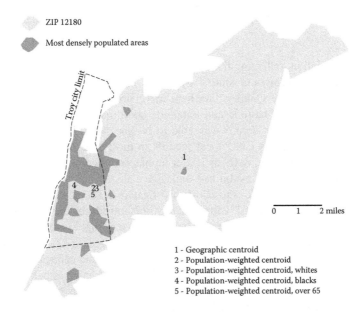

FIGURE 5.2 Centroid locations for ZIP code 12180 (Troy, New York).

TABLE 5.2

GIS Coordinate Quality Codes

Code	Description
00	Coordinates derived from local government-maintained address points, which are based on property parcel locations, not interpolation over a street segment's address range.
01	Coordinates assigned by Global Positioning System (GPS).
02	Coordinates are based on property parcel location.
03	Coordinates are interpolated over the matching street segment's address range.
04	Coordinates are street intersection.
05	Coordinates are midpoint street segments (missing or invalid building number).
06	Coordinates are address ZIP code + 4 centroid.
07	Coordinates are address ZIP code + 2 centroid.
08	Coordinates assigned manually without data linkage.
09	Coordinates are address five-digit ZIP code centroid.
10	Coordinates are point ZIP code of post office box or rural route.
11	Coordinates are centroid of address city (when address ZIP code is unknown or invalid, and there are multiple ZIP codes for the city).
12	Coordinates are centroid of county.
98	Latitude and longitude are assigned, but coordinate quality is unknown.
99	Latitude and longitude are not assigned, but geocoding was attempted; unable to assign coordinates based on available information.
Blank	Gis coordinate quality not coded.

also exhibit variation, reflecting the concentration of blacks in the city of Troy and, to a lesser degree, of seniors in south Troy.

The GIS Coordinate Quality data item in version 11 of the NAACCR layout facilitates the storage of latitude and longitude coordinates for every case record, regardless of whether the record was able to be geocoded (Table 5.2). Although many codes appear in this table, most records in most situations would receive a 03 (for matched records), or an 09 or 10 (for unmatched records), because nearly all cancer case records contain a valid five-digit ZIP code.

One intention of this code is to allow investigators to select just the records that meet a desired quality standard. Unfortunately, this introduces the problem of geographic selection bias discussed here. Another danger is that low-quality geocodes will be inappropriately included in an analysis, despite the GIS Coordinate Quality code. For example, imagine cases assigned to the geographic centroid of ZIP code 12180, with a GIS Coordinate Quality code of 09 but then treated as belonging to the census block group in which the centroid happened to fall. This block group is in a mainly rural area with some encroaching large new homes; it has a poverty rate about half that of the entire ZIP code and a median household income 57% higher, and thus it is not typical of the ZIP code as a whole. If there are enough such cases, then there could be an impact on the analysis — including the possibility of identifying the block group as a cluster or outlier. Partly for this reason, many registries are not yet using the optional GIS Coordinate Quality code, avoiding the "double negative" of storing low-quality data in conjunction with a code indicating the data is of low quality.

5.3.3 GEOGRAPHIC IMPUTATION

Geographic imputation refers to the assignment of a geographic location that is reasonable, if not necessarily accurate, given the available geographic and demographic information about a cancer case. The assigned location may be either an area or a point, depending on the type of analysis conducted.

5.3.3.1 Imputing an Area

With area imputation, the goal is to assign a value for one geographic level (e.g., census tract, census block group) based on information from one or more known geographic levels (e.g., ZIP code, county). This is a common problem not only in cancer surveillance but also in science generally, and different disciplines have developed different terminology and methods for dealing with this issue. Gotway and Young refer to the problem collectively as the "change of support problem."[7] In the following discussion, I use the example of obtaining a census tract from a ZIP code because this is a common situation for central cancer registries.

One simple solution to this problem that does not require GIS software is to take each ungeocoded record, identify a similar geocoded record (one with the same county, ZIP code, age, sex, race, or ethnicity), and assign it to the same location. This can be accomplished in statistical or database software by sorting all records by the known geographic and demographic fields, then assigning each ungeocoded record the location of the record preceding it. (It is not quite this simple; because the preceding record could also be ungeocoded, or could be part of a different stratum, additional conditions must be specified.)

One limitation of this method is that cases will have somewhat of a tendency to cluster. Figure 5.3 again shows ZIP code 12180, which overlaps all or part of 20 different census tracts (for clarity, the tracts are labeled sequentially rather than with their official six-digit tract number). The white and black asterisks denote the tracts where white and black men, respectively, have been diagnosed with prostate cancer over a recent time period. Using this imputation method, an ungeocoded case with black race could be assigned to 1 of only 9 possible tracts, while a case with white race could be assigned to 1 of only 10 possible tracts, even though men of both races live in every tract. This limitation could be overcome with a sufficiently large number of cases (e.g., all male cancers could have been used, not just prostate cancers), but this could in turn be negated if additional strata were added (e.g., if Asians, Hispanics, and 10-year age groups were considered).

An alternative is to use what is known as *areal interpolation*.[8] This GIS-based solution considers all of the possible geographic areas to which a case could be imputed, weighted by area or population. Continuing with the Troy area example, consider tracts 3 and 4 in greater detail. The population of tract 3 is about 2200, and

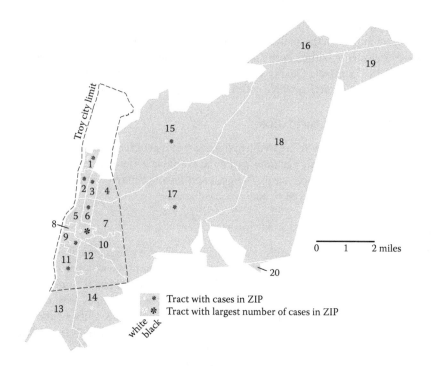

FIGURE 5.3 Imputation of case locations using known locations of other cases.

the population of tract 4 is about 3400, meaning that a case would be more likely to be imputed into tract 4. However, tract 3 falls almost entirely within the 12180 ZIP code; only about one-quarter of tract 4 does. Adjusting the populations by area yields an effective population of 2000 for tract 3 and only 900 for tract 4, making tract 3 a more likely imputed location (Figure 5.4a).

This approach assumes that the population density is uniform within census tracts. In fact, Troy's largest park falls within tract 4 and accounts for much of its area. If block-level populations (the smallest unit for which the Census Bureau publishes data) are considered instead, then the populations of tracts 3 and 4 within the 12180 ZIP are nearly equal (Figure 5.4b). If a person is known to be black, however, then tract 3 is much more likely to be selected (Figure 5.4c). In this example, I have treated the census blocks as points (by using block centroids), meaning that the population of a census block was counted as either entirely within or entirely without the 12180 area. It would have been possible to refine the results further by applying areal interpolation to the census blocks themselves (Figure 5.4d) or by making use of street and road locations.[9] This may all sound complex, but the GIS programming is straightforward.

In this example, there were 20 candidate tracts, meaning that the chance of actually imputing the correct tract was fairly low. Fortuitously, in very rural areas where geocoding rates are lowest, there are often as few as only 1 or 2 candidates. This is because census tracts are designed to have an average population of 4000, but a rural post office may serve fewer than 1000 people. Misclassification is also less of a

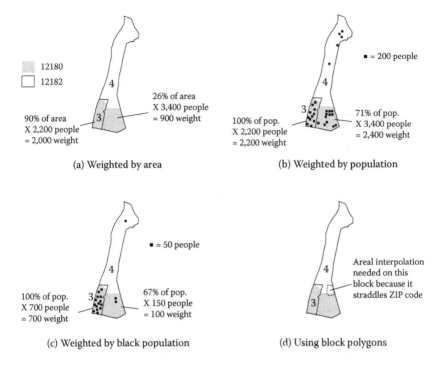

(a) Weighted by area

(b) Weighted by population

(c) Weighted by black population

(d) Using block polygons

FIGURE 5.4 Imputation of case locations using areal interpolation.

concern in rural areas because they tend to be more demographically homogeneous than urban areas.

Still, this begs the question — if imputation is such an uncertain venture, then why not just retain the ZIP code characteristics for the ungeocoded cases and try to do some type of mixed-level spatial analysis in which most of the data are at the census tract level and some are at the ZIP code level? This could work in some situations, but many spatial methods do not work this way — many require that every case must fall within a geographic area, and that geographic areas must touch but not overlap.

5.3.3.2 Imputing a Point

Instead of imputing an area, it might be desirable to try to impute actual latitude and longitude coordinates for an ungeocoded case. Whether this is a useful endeavor depends on whether these coordinates are more analytically useful than the coordinates of the best available centroid, which is typically the ZIP code centroid.

Imputing a point location is not much different from imputing an area location. Simply take all of the nonzero population census blocks and randomly select one, with the selection probability weighted by the population. So, if a ZIP code contains 200 blocks and a total population of 5000, then the chance of selection of a specific block with a population of 100 is 0.02 (1 in 50). Next, assign the coordinates of the centroid of the selected block to the case. As a further level of sophistication, one could assign a random location within the block (although the advantages of this extra step are unclear). To do this, randomly select latitude and longitude values falling within the block's bounding rectangle and then test whether it falls into the block polygon. If it does not, then generate new latitude and longitude values until the condition is met. The block-level populations can be stratified by age, sex, race, or ethnicity. Note that the 2000 census reported counts for those reporting more than one race and those reporting "other" race; for the purposes of imputation, it is easiest to ignore these counts.

Assigning point locations in this manner has the advantage of allowing the cases to be aggregated into any geographic unit for which boundary files exist. Suppose, for example, that case counts are needed by census tract, block group, school district, and city precinct. This would require four separate area imputations, which would be cumbersome. If point locations were imputed instead, then there would only need to be one imputation, and the cases could then be aggregated into each of the four different geographic areas using a simple GIS operation.

For point-based analyses, imputing point locations seems to achieve similar results as using centroids. For example, imagine a distance-to-treatment study in which actual driving distance to the nearest treatment facility is the primary variable of interest and imagine a ZIP code with 10 ungeocoded cases. The cases could all be assigned to the population-weighted centroid location, or they could be assigned imputed locations throughout the ZIP code. The overall average driving distance should be the same because the average location of the 10 scattered cases will correspond to the location of the population-weighted centroid, excepting random error. The analysis using the imputed cases will have greater variance and so is more conservative. Imputing point locations has the additional advantage of not creating artificial clusters at centroid locations. Instead, it biases against finding clusters at the sub-ZIP code level, which is again conservative.

In summary, geographic imputation appears to offer some advantages and no serious drawbacks compared with the alternatives of excluding ungeocoded cases from an analysis or placing them at the best-available centroid (usually the ZIP code centroid). However, formal evaluation of these methods using large data sets has yet to be performed. Members of the NAACCR GIS committee are actively investigating this topic with the hope of providing clearer guidance, and possibly the development of helpful software tools, in the years ahead. As an example of how such a software tool might work, a researcher could submit an input file of ungeocoded records containing county, ZIP code, age, sex, race, or ethnicity and receive a set of imputed geocodes in return. (If desired, the sensitivity of the analytical results to the imputation could be checked by generating multiple sets of imputed geocodes rather than just one.)

When considering imputation methods, it is important to retain a commonsense perspective. In the course of writing this section, I took 20 recent ungeocoded cases from ZIP code 12180 (including all cancer sites, not just prostate cancer) and tracked down their residential addresses using all of the available resources at my disposal. Nearly all were located outside the city of Troy, primarily in recently constructed subdivisions, with several in a recently constructed retirement home. Thus, no imputation method based on 2000 census data would have fared well because the critical factor was not where people were actually living in 2000, but where they were going to be living in the future. One could theoretically incorporate information on pending housing starts, condo conversions, and senior housing construction for every town and city, but obtaining this information would be far more labor intensive than just manually geocoding the cases.

5.4 SUMMARY AND CONCLUSIONS

This chapter has presented a variety of ways to reduce the number of ungeocoded records in a data set, ranging from simple to complex. Past empirical studies have shown that, given sufficient time and resources, just about everyone can be assigned a location. While it may not be practical to track down the most difficult cases, neither is it justifiable to exclude significant shares of cases from a study sample. An approximate location is better than no location at all, and virtually all cancer case records at least come with a useable ZIP code. Depending on the type of analysis being performed, assigning cases to a ZIP code centroid may suffice. But if placing multiple cases in the same arbitrary point location poses a problem, then geographic imputation is a practical alternative. The development and use of techniques for handling missing data have a long tradition in epidemiology;[10] it is time to extend this rigorousness to the spatial realm.

REFERENCES

1. Boscoe FP, Kielb CL, Schymura MJ, Bolani TM. Assessing and improving census tract completeness. *Journal of Registry Management* 29(4): 117–120, 2002.
2. United States Postal Service. Postal Addressing Standards (Publication 28). Washington, DC: United States Postal Service, 2006. http://pe.usps.com/cpim/ftp/pubs/pub28/pub28.pdf. (accessed July 11, 2007)
3. Havener L, Hultstrom D, eds. *Standards for Cancer Registries Volume 2: Data Standards and Data Dictionary*, 10th ed., version 11. Springfield, IL: North American Association of Central Cancer Registries, November 2004.
4. Newcombe HB. *Handbook of Record Linkage: Methods for Health and Statistical Studies, Administration, and Business.* Oxford: Oxford University Press, 1988.
5. Gomatam S, Carter R, Ariet M, Mitchell G. An empirical comparison of record linkage procedures. *Statistics in Medicine* 21: 1485–1496, 2002.
6. McElroy JA, Remington PL, Trentham-Dietz A, Robert SA, Newcomb PA. Geocoding addresses from a large population-based study: lessons learned. *Epidemiology* 14: 399–407, 2003.
7. Gotway CA, Young LJ. Combining incompatible spatial data. *Journal of the American Statistical Association* 97: 632–648, 2002.
8. Flowerdew R, Green M. Developments in areal interpolation methods and GIS. *Annals of Regional Science* 26: 67–78, 1992.
9. Reibel M, Bufalino ME. Street-weighted interpolation techniques for demographic count estimation in incompatible zone systems. *Environment and Planning A* 37: 127–139, 2005.
10. Donders AR, van der Heijden GJ, Stijnen T, Moons KG. Review: A gentle introduction to imputation of missing values. *Journal of Clinical Epidemiology* 59(10): 1087–1091, 2006.

6 Geocoding Practices in Cancer Registries

Toshi Abe and David Stinchcomb

CONTENTS

6.1 INTRODUCTION

Central cancer registries in North America routinely collect information on the residential address of each person diagnosed with cancer. The residential address at the time the patient was diagnosed with cancer and the current residential address are both collected for differing purposes. The address at time of diagnosis is used by epidemiologists for a variety of purposes, such as cancer cluster investigations and descriptive epidemiological reports to show the geographical distribution of cancer and cancer trends over time. The current residential address is used primarily for patient follow-up activities.

    This chapter first describes standards for cancer registry address data. The geocoding practices of a specific registry (the New Jersey State Cancer Registry, NJSCR) are then presented in detail, followed by a review of practices in four other state and local cancer registries to show some of the variations in geocoding practices among cancer registries. Next, we summarize the results of a survey of geocoding practices in 46 state, local, and provincial cancer registries in the United States and Canada. This is followed by a discussion of positional accuracy issues and their impact on cancer registries. We conclude with a brief discussion of future directions in cancer registry geocoding.

6.2   CANCER REGISTRY ADDRESS DATA STANDARDS

Addresses (as well as other demographic and cancer-related data on the patient) are collected and coded following standards that are developed principally by the North American Association of Central Cancer Registries (NAACCR); the Surveillance, Epidemiology, and End Results (SEER) Program of the National Cancer Institute (NCI); and the American College of Surgeons Commission on Cancer (CoC). A compilation of these standards may be found in the NAACCR series *Standards for Cancer Registries, Volumes 1–5* (available at http://www.naaccr.org). Volume 2 contains the data dictionary and rules for collecting and coding geographical information about the cancer patient.[1]

The data items currently collected for the patient's residential address at the time of diagnosis include these fields:

- Street number and name, street type, street direction, and apartment number
- Building name, apartment complex name, or facility name (such as nursing home, hospital, or prison)
- City or town name
- State code
- ZIP code
- County code
- Latitude and longitude
- Geographic information system (GIS) coordinate quality field to record the basis on which the latitude and longitudes were assigned
- Two separate census tract fields, the first to record the census tract value for the 1970 through 1990 censuses and the second for the 2000 census tract value
- Census tract certainty field to record the basis on which the census tract was assigned (usually the full street address)
- Census tract block group

Although the patient's current address is also collected by cancer registries, it is the residential address at the time of diagnosis that is usually geoprocessed and used by geographers and epidemiologists to help perform and conduct epidemiological analyses of cancer patterns in the community.

Most cancer registries routinely geocode the address of the patient at diagnosis to obtain the value for the census tract field. The census tract information is required by the SEER Program of the NCI and the Centers for Disease Control and Prevention's (CDC) National Program of Cancer Registries (NPCR). For confidentiality purposes, only the county, state, and census tract fields are sent to the SEER and NPCR programs to meet their data submission requirements.

To meet the census tract field requirement, cancer registries rely on geoprocessing vendor services or perform geoprocessing in-house. In the next two sections, we look at how some specific cancer registries perform this geoprocessing to produce accurately geocoded data for spatial epidemiological analyses.

6.3 GEOCODING PRACTICES IN THE NEW JERSEY STATE CANCER REGISTRY

The NJSCR contains over 1.2 million records of cancer that have been reported by law since 1979, the cancer registry's first full year of operation. Over 80,000 new case reports of cancer are reported annually to the registry. All of these addresses are geocoded by in-house staff who use the commercially available geoprocessing software product Integrity GeoLocator from Ascential Software, Incorporated (Boston, MA).

The Integrity GeoLocator uses probabilistic matching methods (see chapter 5) to link street address data to an enhanced GDT (Geographic Data Technologies) street reference file, which is updated by the company on a regular basis. Embedded in the product are powerful tools to condition and standardize the address data and well-tested matching software to perform the actual geocoding. These data-standardizing and data-matching tools are Superstan and Supermatch, respectively, which were originally marketed as AutoStan and AutoMatch.

6.3.1 DATA CLEANSING AND ADDRESS STANDARDIZATION

The NJSCR regularly submits batches of address data to the Integrity GeoLocator for processing. The steps performed in this process are:

1. Cleansing and standardization of address data elements
2. Matching the street address to a street reference file
3. Returning successfully geocoded and standardized data elements; ungeocodeable address records are also returned for review

Cleansing and standardization help ensure that address elements conform to U.S. Postal Service (USPS) standards and that they meet Coding Accuracy Support System (CASS) certification rules. Some of the typical data-cleansing and address standardization problems that the system resolves are as follows:

- Misspelled street and city or town names are corrected.
  - CHURSH ST becomes CHURCH ST
  - MONTIVILLE, NJ becomes MONTVILLE, NJ
- Standards for numerical street names are applied.
  - THIRD STREET becomes 3RD ST
- Standard abbreviations are assigned.
  - LANE becomes LN
  - N, S, E, and W replace the street directions North, South, East, and West.

- Missing, invalid, or incorrect ZIP codes are corrected and reassigned for the match.
  - Paterson, NJ 07522 with an incorrect ZIP is standardized to Paterson, NJ 07506

One danger of automated data cleansing and standardizing is the incorrect substitutions of address data elements. For example, the NJSCR once found, with a different standardizing product, that an incomplete street address TH STREET was standardized to THOMAS ST. With the Integrity GeoLocator, the NJSCR recently saw the street address 999 UNKNOWN changed to 999 UNIONHILL. One way to guard against incorrect standardization of data is to regularly perform quality control assessments of the results. For example, with the Integrity GeoLocator it is helpful to review those probabilistic match scores with low scores (i.e., scores under 15).

6.3.2 GEOCODED RESULTS

The NJSCR links the CASS-certified addresses to the street reference file through the Integrity GeoLocator system's Supermatch component. A number of geocoded elements are returned to the user for each successful match; addresses that fail the CASS certification process are returned to the user for manual review or correction. The results returned from the Integrity GeoLocator process include these appended fields:

- Low and high address ranges for the left and right sides of streets
- Standardized street names
- Standardized city names
- Standardized Federal information processing standards (FIPS) county codes (left and right values)
- Standardized five-digit ZIP postal codes
- Census tract codes (2000 census definitions, left and right values)
- Census block values (left and right)
- Latitude and longitude coordinates
- GeoLocator match indicator: Indicates whether the match was an exact street address match, a street segment match (the street number was out of range), a street intersection match, or a postal ZIP code match or if no match was found; also indicates whether the match was to a single street or to multiple streets
- Probabilistic weighted match scores for each street address-level match

With accurate street address data, the expectation is that reasonably accurate latitude and longitude coordinates will be returned from the geocoding process. Accurate coordinates allow one to more truly locate the patient's residence address on a map, which ensures that the assignment of county and subcounty levels is more likely to be correct. The NJSCR has found that a small percentage of county codes change as a result of the geocoding process. The original county code is often set based on the ZIP code. The registry has identified 83 postal ZIP codes in which the ZIP code boundary crosses county lines. For example, Princeton, New Jersey, has a postal ZIP code, 08540, that is used by municipalities in the counties of Mercer, Middlesex, and Somerset. County codes in these ZIP codes can be more accurately assigned based on the latitude and longitude determined from geocoding.

6.3.3 Manual Review and Address Correction Problems

Addresses that fail to be CASS certified are returned for further review or correction. In practice, the Integrity GeoLocator returns about 85% of submitted addresses with geocodes that match to an exact street address. Another 6% to 7% of addresses only match to a ZIP code level. The remaining addresses require manual review and are reviewed along with the addresses that were not CASS certified. Then, addresses that are manually corrected are resubmitted for geoprocessing.

The NJSCR's experience with the Integrity GeoLocator shows that the following types of address problems are likely to require manual intervention:

- Addresses entered with no spaces between elements
  - 101MAINST
- Box numbers followed by a street name
  - BOX 595 ROCKWELL RD
- Street addresses containing an institutional name
  - VETERANS HOME ONE VALLEY RD
- Local names that are not in the street reference file
  - CONVENT STATION, NJ, a local name within Morristown, NJ, is missing from the street reference file.
- Postal ZIP codes that have changed
  - Once the updated ZIP code is applied, exact street address matches are found. For example, in New Jersey, parts of ZIP code 08733 changed to 08759.
  - To decrease the number of cases not geocoded because of a change in ZIP code, the NJSCR reviewed all of the issues of the USPS *Postal Bulletin* between 1995 and 2005 and documented all New Jersey ZIP code changes. The *Postal Bulletin* is published monthly by the USPS and provides a list of all the nationwide ZIP code changes (see http://www.usps.com/cpim/ftp/bulletin/pb.htm).
- Two possible street numbers with a match when one of the numbers is used
  - 650 10 MAIN ST may yield a match using 10 MAIN ST but not 650 MAIN ST.

A geographer at the New York State Department of Health, working with large address files, has written a useful computer program that automatically corrects problematic street addresses. Addresses that fail to match a street reference file are processed by this program to fix some commonly occurring problems. The program applies the following changes to see if the resulting address can be successfully geocoded:

- Strip hyphens and other special characters such as !, @, #, $, ^, &, and * from the address.
- If the first word in the street starts with RD, then delete it.
  - RD2 GANNON RD becomes GANNON RD.
- If the first word contains a number and a letter, then delete the letter.
  - 500B N MAIN ST becomes 500 N MAIN ST.
- If the second word is a single letter, then delete it.
  - 500 B N MAIN ST becomes 500 N MAIN ST.

- If the first letter in a word is N, S, E, or W, then follow it with a space.
  - 14 NMANNING BLVD becomes 14 N MANNING BLVD.
- If the first letters in a word are NO or SO, then follow them with a space.
  - 14 NOMANNING BLVD becomes 14 NO MANNING BLVD.
- If an address does not contain RR, BOX, and so on, then remove all words that precede the number.
  - CLOVER REST HOME 28 WASHINGTON ST becomes 28 WASHINGTON ST.
  - c/o JIM SMITH 399 JEFFERSON ST becomes 399 JEFFERSON ST.

To facilitate geocoding when only facility names are given, as in the case of Clover Rest Home, it is also helpful to maintain a database of addresses for nursing homes, hospitals, apartment buildings, and public housing units.

6.3.4 Attainable Geocoding Match Rates

The NJSCR in the 1980s and 1990s relied on commercial vendors to perform geocoding operations. The goal was to obtain the census tract for each address record. At best, however, the NJSCR found that the commercial vendors were able to find an exact street-level match about 70% of the time. The major problem preventing the registry from obtaining higher results was the quality of the address data, which was badly in need of cleaning. The task of correcting the remaining addresses can be time consuming. For smaller cancer registries, manually correcting difficult-to-geocode addresses might be manageable, but for medium- to large-size registries, which collect up to 80,000 or more cancer reports annually, computer software solutions are preferred.

Using the Integrity system, with its powerful address-standardizing modules Superstan and Supermatch, the NJSCR has been able to obtain street-level matches of 85% or better on the first pass of the data. With additional manual review of the unmatched records, the NJSCR is usually able to improve its street-level match rate to about 92%. An additional 6% to 7% of the address data matches to the ZIP code level, which leaves less than 2% of the data ungeocodeable. (These figures exclude cases for which the source of information is only from a death certificate.) Thus, by relying on the Integrity system for the bulk of its geocoding needs, the NJSCR is now able to match over 90% of its address data to the census tract matched to a street address.

For more information on the subject of street reference files and geocoding, see the excellent discussion in the NAACCR publication, *Using Geographic Information Systems Technology in the Collection, Analysis, and Presentation of Cancer Registry Data: A Handbook of Basic Practices*, available from the NAACCR GIS Committee Web site at http://www.naaccr.org/gis.[2]

6.3.5 Interactive Geocoding Services

For a variety of reasons, the automated geoprocessing performed by the Integrity GeoLocator sometimes fails to geocode addresses that appear to have all necessary address components in place. To help solve this problem, the NJSCR is currently setting up an interactive geocoding service using ArcView 9.x that will allow a geocoding clerk to work with street address data that failed to geocode with the automated

Integrity process. Once trained, the clerk should be able to process approximately 150 addresses per hour. Besides working with addresses that failed to geocode, the clerk will be given address data that were previously geocoded to the ZIP code centroid. The NJSCR hopes to be able to convert these ZIP code matches to street address-level matches. Approximately 70,000 records are eligible for this project.

6.4 GEOCODING PRACTICES IN OTHER REGISTRIES

In this section, we briefly describe geocoding practices in four other cancer registries, focusing on the unique aspects of each. Different basic geocoding software products and methods are used in each registry. In addition, Arizona has defined a set of geographic areas between the county and the census tract that is used for cancer data reporting. In Detroit, the cancer registry does much of its basic geocoding via simple table matches rather than using specialized geocoding software, and it collaborates with a nearby research center when more detailed geographic information is needed. North Carolina makes extensive use of parcel and address data from local governments and takes an active role in improving the quality of address data in the state. Alaska's unique geography not only presents special challenges but also allows for interesting solutions that could be applied in other sparsely populated areas.

6.4.1 The Arizona Cancer Registry

In Arizona, a state with large counties and a rapidly growing population, a stable area of analysis was needed to provide rates for communities at a scale smaller than county level while maintaining a population large enough to support analysis. The Arizona Department of Health Services (ADHS) has developed Community Health Analysis Areas (CHAAs) to represent communities. All levels of management within ADHS were briefed about the CHAA development as the CHAA design took shape. The Environmental Systems Research Institute (ESRI)'s ArcGIS was used to create the CHAAs. The development of the CHAAs was based on areas originally devised to evaluate primary medical care (primary care areas or PCAs). Although CHAAs were developed from PCAs, the aims of the two analysis areas were not the same. After the CHAAs were completed, the program responsible for the PCA analysis was consulted to ensure that the program would not interfere with the PCA mission and purpose. Both PCAs and CHAAs used 2000 census block groups to create the areas of analysis. CHAAs give the user the ability to aggregate any data from the block group level up to the CHAA level in analysis.

The Arizona Cancer Registry geocodes its own cases. Addresses are first run through a commercial geocoding package (Centrus) to standardize and geocode most cases. Cases that cannot be geocoded to the address level are manually reviewed. Cases with incorrect addresses are corrected and rerun through Centrus. Cases with post office boxes or rural addresses are run through an ArcView composite geocoding service that consists of a series of programs that geocode to the smallest area possible. Rules for inclusion in each level of geography were devised to ensure the greatest possible accuracy supported by the available data. The Arizona Cancer Registry codes latitude, longitude, census tract, block group, county, and CHAA from this geocoding process.

6.4.2 THE METROPOLITAN DETROIT CANCER SURVEILLANCE SYSTEM

The Metropolitan Detroit Cancer Surveillance System (MDCSS) does not use special geocoding software. Instead, it uses an in-house procedure to match residential information at time of cancer diagnosis with census tract. In this procedure, the patient's address at diagnosis is recorded in separate fields (street number, street direction, ZIP code, and county code), which are then matched with the 2000 Topologically Integrated Geographic Encoding and Referencing (TIGER) system line files that contain data on census tract for each street segment.

Addresses that fail to geocode are manually reviewed by staff using Bresser's Cross-index Directory, a name and street address cross reference available for most of Michigan and parts of Indiana, Wisconsin, and Florida (http://www.bressers. com). Similar local street and address reference products are available from local companies in many other large urban areas and can be a useful source for up-to-date street and address information.

For special projects, the MDCSS works collaboratively with the Michigan Metropolitan Information Center at Wayne State University, which is able to provide geocodes to the census block group level. Latitude and longitude coordinates are not currently stored by the MDCSS, although coordinates are used for some special studies.

6.4.3 THE NORTH CAROLINA CENTRAL CANCER REGISTRY

The North Carolina Central Cancer Registry (NCCCR) uses in-house staff to perform all of its geoprocessing. They batch match all records, which number about 500,000 since 1990. About 35,000 new records are added annually. The NCCCR batch matching criteria is 98% minimum match score on all address components and zone items. The software products used are ArcGIS 9x, MS Access, Oracle, and DataFlux. Their batch geocode success rate is 64% statewide, and that figure discounts addresses that are not geocodeable, such as post office boxes.

Reference data sources employed are pre-2004 GDT and 2004 TeleAtlas street centerline files, shape files of previously geocoded addresses, and local government-maintained parcel and address point files. Local government-maintained data are available for all or part of about 60% of the counties in North Carolina. The NCCCR is actively involved in statewide GIS groups and lobbies for uniform standards for local government parcel and address point data, which would help reduce geographical data maintenance activities.

At NCCCR, none of the geocodes can have an uncertain census block group. Thus, ZIP codes or other centroids with bounding polygons that are not exactly contiguous with census enumeration polygons are used. NCCCR geocodes to streets contained in a census block group, interpolated street positions, intersections, and centroids or other points within residential parcels.

NCCCR uses Semaphore Corporation's ZP4 product to validate addresses prior to geocoding. NCCCR also uses local government-maintained address points to identify addresses with incorrect USPS ZIP + 4 county codes. NCCCR has agreements with the two USPS Address Management Offices in the state such that, when NCCCR identifies addresses more than 2000 feet from a county border with ZIP + 4 county codes that are incorrect, NCCCR sends the correct information to the appropriate USPS Address Management Office, where updates are made to the ZIP + 4 database for the following month's release.

Interactive (manual) geocoding is also employed, with the degree of success varying by county. NCCCR stores information about each manually geocoded address in metadata. These metadata are then available if the same or a similar address occurs again. At the time of interactive processing, NCCCR records in the metadata information such as whether the problem was with the geocode source or the address, whether the address required editing for a match, and whether the address was derived from non-NCCCR data. An old/new comparison program is run to help automate the process of matching old geocodes and metadata with recurrent addresses and their variants. In this way, previously rejected addresses pass on their metadata to incoming addresses.

A challenge facing North Carolina is that, in its rural counties, upward of 60% have post office boxes for addresses, which makes it difficult to perform spatial analyses in these areas. Attempts are under way to gain access to the address data from the state's Division of Motor Vehicles to update/verify post office box addresses. In the meantime, cluster investigations in these areas are treated as special cases. For those post office boxes that cannot be geocoded, the cases are assigned street addresses by linking to county property tax databases via identification fields in the cancer record, such as first, middle, and last name.

6.4.4 THE ALASKA CANCER REGISTRY

Geocoding at the Alaska Cancer Registry is in its infancy. Staffing is limited, but the geography of this state helps to compensate for scarce geocoding resources. There are only 348 towns in Alaska, and just 10 of them have more than one census tract. Also, most towns are fairly small, and all have only one county FIPS code. To assign census tracts correctly, Alaska Cancer Registry staff use a Microsoft Access table of town names, county FIPS codes, and census tract codes. Each cancer patient's address is matched to this census tract table simply on the basis of the town name. For those towns with more than one census tract, the Alaska Cancer Registry currently codes these census tracts as 999999. The Alaska Cancer Registry uses MapInfo Professional for GIS work and has MapInfo MapMarker for geocoding, although it has not yet been utilized for cancer registry data. The Alaska Cancer Registry plans to start using MapMarker in the near future to replace the unknown census tract entries with real values.

An interesting address issue for geocoding in Alaska is that many small towns do not have street addresses, so all residents of such towns use post office boxes. For geocoding purposes, these people would be represented as points at the town centroid. Because these towns have only one census tract, it is straightforward to assign this value to each patient's address. Accurate assignment of latitude and longitude, however, is not possible for these cases.

6.5 SURVEY OF REGISTRY GEOCODING PRACTICES

In spring and summer of 2005, the NAACCR GIS Committee conducted a survey of GIS practices among 72 NAACCR member cancer registries. A total of 46 registries responded from the United States and Canada, the vast majority (41) state-level central

TABLE 6.1

Usage of Alternative Geocoding Methods (Percentage of Use by Registries Performing Geocoding)

Alternative Geocoding Method	Usage (%)
Remove nongeocodable addresses prior to geocoding	54
Standardize the address	70
Use text substitution for common address variants	46
Do automated match using more than one data source	27
Allow matches to large-area centroids (such as ZIP codes)	78
Use manual/interactive geocoding for unmatched records	57
Reuse previous geocodes for new records with the same address	18

cancer registries in the United States. Of the responding registries, 82% reported that they geocode the address at diagnosis.

Of the registries performing geocoding, it was fairly evenly divided between those who use geocoding services from commercial vendors (33%), those who perform the geocoding within the cancer registry (28%), and those who use geocoding services provided by another division within their organization (37%). Some registries reported using various combinations of these methods.

There is wide variety in the number of records geocoded each year, which reflects the wide range of populations covered by the various registries. On average, the number of addresses run through the geocoding process is about 1.7 times the annual caseload because of both the resubmission of record batches after address editing and the geocoding of data from prior years. Some form of address cleaning is performed by 83% of the geocoding registries. Of the addresses submitted for geocoding, an average of 84% are matched in batch mode, and a total of 93% are geocoded by either batch or manual geocoding.

Table 6.1 provides a summary of the usage of various alternative methods in the geocoding process.

Registries report using a wide variety of supplemental address data to update, correct, or confirm address information. These include birth and death certificate data, voter registration records, motor vehicle registration records, driver's license data, Medicare and Medicaid data, day care records, other disease registry information, hospital information systems data, and tribal health services data.

6.6 ACCURACY OF THE GEOCODE

The success of the geocoding process is most often measured in terms of the *match rate*, the percentage of cases that were successfully geocoded. Equally important is the *positional accuracy* of the geocode, that is, how close the estimated location is to the true location. For cancer registries, the main concern is the impact of geocoding location errors on subsequent use of the locational information. Such errors include classification errors (cancer cases assigned to the wrong county or associated with an incorrect environmental exposure estimate), errors in mapping cancer rates, and the incorrect identification or location of cancer clusters.

Several articles have reported on the accuracy of geocoded data and the geocoding process. In an article by Yang et al.[3] the researchers concluded that differences in preprocessing of address data elements accounted for a large percentage of the discrepancies in the geocoded results of three different geoprocessing software packages. Krieger et al.[4] found similar inaccuracies among four different commercial geocoding firms. Whitsel et al.[5] reported on the accuracy and repeatability of commercial geocoding vendors. Boscoe et al.[6] reported on the most common reasons why addresses fail to geocode in an automated geocoding process.

In addition, a number of articles have reported the results of comparisons of geocoded positions with "true" locations. In these studies, true locations were determined by either use of Global Positioning System (GPS) devices or analysis of aerial imagery. The primary measure of interest was the distance between the geocoded location and the true location. The studies also evaluated angular differences, changes in positional error over time, and differences between geocoding methods. Here, we summarize the results from three such studies.

Bonner et al.[7] compared 200 addresses in western New York State from a case-control study. True locations were determined using a GPS device. They compared positional error for urban and rural addresses; *urban* was defined as within the city limits of a major city. They found median errors of 32 meters for urban addresses and 52 meters for rural addresses (see Table 6.2 for a summary). The study found similar errors for cases and controls. The data included residential histories from 1930 to 2000, and the analysis did not show a significant difference on the positional error across decades.

TABLE 6.2
Summary of Geocoding Positional Error (in meters)

	Bonner et al. (2003)	Cayo & Talbot (2003)[a]	Ward et al. (2005)
Urban/Town			
Median	32	38	56
75th percentile	—	—	92
90th percentile	37	96	—
Mean	96	58	77
Max	1,551	1,088	687
Rural/Nonurban			
Median	52	201	88
75th percentile	—	—	254
90th percentile	61	1,544	—
Mean	129	614	210
Max	2,552	18,742	1,731

[a] Suburban classification results are not shown.

Cayo and Talbot[8] evaluated 3000 addresses from property tax databases in four counties in the Albany, New York, area. True locations were derived primarily from aerial imagery, with a GPS used in ambiguous cases. They compared errors for urban, suburban, and rural areas, as classified by population density. They found a median error of 38 meters for urban addresses, 78 meters for suburban addresses, and 201 meters for rural addresses. They found much less positional error when using the centroids of the parcels from the property tax databases for geocoding rather than interpolating from street segment matches. They also found that errors did not have much angular differentiation (i.e., errors were not larger or smaller in any one direction).

Ward et al.[9] evaluated the positional accuracy of 234 addresses from 43 counties in south-central Iowa as part of a case-control study of pesticide exposure. True locations were taken from a GPS device. They evaluated error within the incorporated areas of towns with error outside towns. They found median errors of 56 meters for addresses in towns and 88 meters for addresses outside towns. They found the commercial vendor did not have less positional error than in-house geocoding overall and had generally greater errors in the rural areas. They noted that pesticide exposure classification was affected by geocoding errors for 100-meter buffers but not for larger buffer sizes.

Table 6.2 summarizes the results of these three studies. Note that the definitions of urban and rural areas were not consistent between studies, and the differing definitions may account for some of the differences between the results.

All three studies found greater errors in rural areas than in more urban areas, probably because of both the denser street networks and more complete and up-to-date street databases available in urban areas. The fact that the Ward et al. 2005 study in rural Iowa found greater errors overall than the two studies from New York State probably reflects the more rural nature of the study area. The larger rural median error in the Cayo and Talbot study (201 meters) is likely partly because of the separate classification of suburban addresses.[8] Cayo and Talbot found the largest 90th percentile and maximum errors, perhaps because of the significantly larger sample size (3000 addresses rather than 200–234 addresses).

Current geocoding processes generally do not provide a positional error estimate in terms of distance. Rather, we have only the type of match (street address, ZIP + 4, ZIP + 2, ZIP, etc.) to use to decide whether the degree of accuracy is adequate for a particular study. These match types are captured in the GIS Coordinate Quality field of the standard NAACCR data record. Current valid values for this field were given in Table 5.2.

To understand better how the match type relates to classification errors, Bushhouse et al.[10] analyzed the percentage of correct census tract assignment by geocoding match type for a set of cancer registry addresses in different areas of Minnesota. They found that street address-level matches generally received the correct census tract assignment in all areas — well over 95%. ZIP + 2 matches performed well in some areas, but there was a large proportion of incorrect census tract assignments in one area. ZIP code-level matches performed poorly in all areas, with less than 80% correct census tract matches. These results suggest that it may be risky to use ZIP-level geocode locations in a study that depends on correct census tract assignments, for example, to study health disparities based on neighborhood socio-economic factors.

In addition to classification errors, there are other ways in which geocoding accuracy can affect epidemiological studies. Geocoding errors can result in changes to maps of disease rates and can modify the spatial location of disease clusters. For example, Oliver et al.[11] reported a significant shift in the location of prostate cancer clusters in Virginia primarily because of incomplete geocoding in the rural areas of Virginia.

At this time, geocoding accuracy research provides a still somewhat incomplete picture. For more complete understanding, we need studies of positional accuracy in other parts of the country. We also need further studies of the relationship between geocoding match type and positional accuracy and of the impact of positional errors on epidemiological studies, including maps and cluster studies. To partially address these needs, the NCI has funded three studies on the accuracy of the geocoded data in cancer registries. Registries in Detroit, Atlanta (which includes a set of rural counties in Georgia), and the Seattle-Puget Sound area were selected for this study. The areas are sufficiently diverse to allow for both urban and rural areas to be measured for the accuracy of their geocoded cancer registry data. Researchers will evaluate the impact of geocoding accuracy on epidemiological analysis, including maps and cluster identification. Results from these studies are expected in the near future.

6.7 THE FUTURE OF GEOCODING IN CANCER REGISTRIES

Currently, there are a number of geocoding improvements on the horizon for cancer registries. These involve improvements in the data sources, improvements to the geocoding process itself, and improvements in the output data.

There is a general desire to move from the periodic batch geocoding of thousands of records to more real-time geocoding when case records first enter the registry or even when the residence address information is initially recorded by the service provider. Many of the new generation of registry data management systems have plans to include geocoding processing during standard registry record-processing steps. This will allow early identification of errors in the input address fields. Also, several registries are working to provide address verification and standardization software to their local service providers to allow residence addresses to be checked when the data are first entered. This will allow corrections to be made at the local level and could greatly improve the quality of the residence address information.

Another trend is to move from matching street segments and the linear interpolation of the location to full matching of the entire address with point-level location information. For example, as seen here, the parcel-level data sources used by the NCCCR are matched by the full address (street number as well as street name) and provide a specific point location (usually the centroid of the parcel). Also, many of the major geocoding source data vendors are starting to provide point-level address data, usually based on county parcel databases as well as the traditional street segment data. The use of point-level address data will greatly improve the positional accuracy of the geocoding results.

Most registries routinely geocode a single address for each case: the residence address at the time of diagnosis. There is a growing interest in the geographic location over time. Most cancers have a long latency period, some as long as 10–20 years. A residential history of cancer patients will be needed to study the impact of their geographic location over time, and this will involve geocoding multiple addresses for each case. Also, the increased interest in cancer survivorship issues brings potential analytic value to the current geographic location of the patient. Most registries record the current address of the patient for follow-up activities and to contact the patient for case-control interview studies. Currently, these addresses are rarely geocoded, and new addresses simply replace previous addresses. There would need to be some fairly major changes to both the current sources of address information and the standard record layout to allow the tracking of residential histories both before and after diagnosis in support of these emerging research areas.

Finally, future improvements can be made in the information recorded about the positional accuracy of a geocode. The current set of GIS coordinate quality values in the standard cancer data record does not provide a quantitative estimate of positional accuracy. Future geocoding software could automatically record a quantitative estimate of the positional accuracy of each geocode based on the size and spatial resolution of the matched data source. These quantitative estimates could then be used to provide a positional "confidence interval" to guide the selection of geocoded records for individual spatial analysis research projects.

ACKNOWLEDGMENTS

We thank the following for their contributions to this section: Frank Boscoe, New York State Cancer Registry; Joanne Harris and Kendra Schwartz, Metropolitan Detroit Cancer Surveillance System; Christian Klaus, North Carolina Central Cancer Registry; Chris Newton, Arizona Cancer Registry; David O'Brien, Alaska Cancer Registry; and Recinda Sherman and Lydia Voti, Florida Cancer Data System.

REFERENCES

1. Hoffenkamp J, Havener L (EDs.). *Standards for Cancer Registries Vol. II: Data Standards and Data Dictionary*, 12th ed. version 11.2, Springfield, IL: North American Association of Central Cancer Registries, April 2007.
2. Wiggins L (Ed.). *Using Geographic Information Systems Technology in the Collection, Analysis, and Presentation of Cancer Registry Data: A Handbook of Basic Practices.* Springfield, IL: North American Association of Central Cancer Registries, October 2002.
3. Yang DH, Bilaver LM, Hayes O, Goerge R. Improving geocoding practices: evaluation of geocoding tools. *J Med Syst,* 28:361–370, 2004.
4. Krieger N, Waterman P, Lemieux K, Zierler S, Hogan J. On the wrong side of the tracts? Evaluating the accuracy of geocoding in public health research. *Am J Public Health,* 91:1114–1116, 2001.
5. Whitsel EA, Rose KM, Wood JL, Henley AC, Duanping L, Heiss G. Accuracy and repeatability of commercial geocoding. *Am J Epidemiol,* 160:1023–1029, 2004.
6. Boscoe F, Kielb CL, Schymura MJ, Bolani TM. Assessing and improving census tract completeness. *J Reg Manag,* 29:117–120, 2002.

7. Bonner MR, Han D, Nie J, Rogerson P, Vena JE, Freudenheim JL. Positional accuracy of geocoded addresses in epidemiologic research. *Epidemiology.* Jul; 14(4):408–12, 2003.

8. Cayo MR, Talbot, TO. Positional error in automated geocoding of residential addresses. *Int J Health Geogr,* 2:10, 2003.

9. Ward MH, Nuckols JR, Giglierano J, Bonner MR, Wolter C, Airola M, Mix W, Colt JS, Hartge P. Positional accuracy of two methods of geocoding. *Epidemiology,* 16:542–547, 2005.

10. Bushhouse S, Larson C, Williams A. Accuracy of vendor geocoding for rural addresses. Paper presented at the NAACCR Annual Meeting, June 11, 2003, Honolulu, Hawaii.

11. Oliver MN, Matthews KA, Siadaty M, Hauck FR, Pickle LW. Geographic bias related to geocoding in epidemiologic studies. *Int J Health Geogr,* 4:29, 2005.

7 Alternative Techniques for Masking Geographic Detail to Protect Privacy

Dale L. Zimmerman, Marc P. Armstrong, and Gerard Rushton

CONTENTS

7.1 INTRODUCTION

The geographic information system (GIS) literature has contributed little to describing technical measures that are designed to protect privacy in a GIS environment. Instead, it has recognized and commented on a variety of ways in which knowledge of the locations of individuals can compromise their privacy and make it difficult to protect the confidentiality of records of individuals in a GIS environment.[1–7] VanWey et al. discussed conflicts between preserving social-spatial data linkages and confidentiality protection.[8]

Point maps of geocoded records that accurately display locations of cancer cases and other health events can compromise confidentiality because they can be used to recover individual addresses through reverse geocoding.[2,9,10] As Rushton et al.

explained, the process of inverse geocoding "first determines an address from the location of each map symbol, then uses it to forge a link to other data sources."[11]

There are a number of different federal and state laws directed at protecting the confidentiality of individually identifiable health information, including that of cancer patients. These laws vary greatly in their specific confidentiality requirements with respect to the use and disclosure of such information. The laws may be applicable to the use and disclosure of geocoded data sets depending on the original source of data and the custodian of the data. In general, there are two main approaches for protecting the confidentiality of geocoded cancer registry data and other individual health data. One approach involves restricting access to geocoded data sets. Thus, organizational entities and individuals holding geocoded data sets may restrict access to geocoded data sets to specifically approved institutions and persons for specifically approved purposes. The other approach involves the deidentification of such data sets prior to their release to researchers or the general public. For a detailed discussion of confidentiality issues and legal requirements to protect the confidentiality of geocoded cancer registry and other health data, see chapter 12, this volume.

Unfortunately, limitations on disclosure of geocoded data directed at confidentiality protection may have a negative impact on the utility of the data for cancer surveillance and research. Armstrong, Rushton, and Zimmerman pointed out that "[t]hough interest in the geographical analysis of disease has increased, there has been very little discussion of practical ways to protect the confidentiality of data while permitting valid analyses."[12]

Wartell and McEwen noted, in the context of permitting researchers to have access to geocoded crime data, that

> Researchers are accustomed to signing agreements to ensure the confidentiality of individuals when analyzing survey data, but such agreements are not prevalent regarding geocoded data. The field has yet to agree on what restrictions should be placed on researchers' use of data that will safeguard confidentiality while enabling researchers to spatially analyze [data using] rigorous methods — methods that ultimately serve the entire criminal justice field.[13]

The same can be said of geocoded health data. One principle that holds promise is that of k-anonymity, which defines k as "the number of people among whom a specified de-identified case cannot be reversely identified."[14]

The subject of this chapter is geographic masking approaches in which confidentiality is afforded by systematically altering the geographic referencing of data so that certain relationships can be investigated without the risk of disclosure of the identity of individuals. Other masking approaches, discussed in this and other chapters, involve aggregating to larger spatial entities than the original geocodes.

7.2 GEOGRAPHIC MASKING APPROACHES

7.2.1 GENERAL FRAMEWORK

A general framework for describing and comparing microdata masking procedures was introduced by Duncan and Pearson and adapted for geographic masking by Armstrong et al.[12,15] In this framework, the true and complete data file is represented by an *n*-by-*p* matrix *X*, of which the *n* rows correspond to individuals and the *p* columns correspond to attributes. We assume that *X* has been stripped of its obvious formal identifiers, such as name and social security number. The objective of the data custodian (the organization holding the protected data) is to release a modified (i.e., masked) version of *X* that preserves the spatial information to a level of precision sufficient for the user's purposes while keeping the disclosure risk below an acceptable level.

For our purposes, it is useful to partition *X* as follows:

$$X = [U, V, W, Z]$$

where *U* and *V* are geographic coordinates, *W* consists of explicit health variables (e.g., presence or absence of a particular health condition), and *Z* contains other relevant attributes such as age, gender, or ambient levels of environmental contamination. Most geographic masks leave *W* and *Z* untouched and replace the original geographic coordinates with a new pair of coordinates obtained through a transformation $g(\cdot)$. The result of such masks is a matrix, $M = [g(U, V), W, Z]$, of the same dimensions as *X*. A few masks result in an *M* matrix of lesser or greater dimensions than *X*.

7.2.2 AGGREGATION

By far the most common geographic masking method is the aggregation of individual-level health information to areal units. Often, the units of aggregation are taken to be preexisting political or administrative entities, for example, counties, census tracts, or ZIP (postal) codes; these units may have the added benefit of having social, demographic, or environmental information available for them that can be used in an analysis. The county is the unit of aggregation most frequently used by national health institutions such as the U.S. Centers for Disease Control and Prevention; smaller areas are typically used by state and local health agencies. To maintain confidentiality at sufficient levels, some organizations place restrictions on the population of the areal unit used for masking; the U.S. National Center for Health Statistics, for example, requires that health information not be reported for geographic units with fewer than 100,000 inhabitants.

Although areal aggregation to political or administrative units is the norm, aggregation may alternatively be performed in more flexible and context-dependent ways that enable researchers to provide health information for areas that are relevant for hypotheses of interest. For example, lung cancer cases could be reported for annular regions centered at an industrial incinerator. Nonconterminous spatial aggregation could even be considered, such as aggregating asthma cases within a county among individuals living within 0.5 mile, 1 mile, 1.5 miles, and so on of concentrated animal feeding operations.

Another, less-common approach to aggregation, known as *point aggregation*, is to use a single location to represent a defined subset of the original locations of health events. For example, areal units of aggregation could be represented by their centroids. Less trivially, locations of health events could be grouped, and all those belonging to the same group could be assigned to a single point using location-allocation algorithms. These algorithms minimize the sum of squares from the original locations to a smaller number of locations, one representing each group.[16]

In terms of the general geographic masking framework, areal aggregation consists of assigning U and V to a set of geographic regions, each element of which is deemed to have sufficient population to protect the confidentiality of individuals. The resulting data matrix is $M = [P, W, Z]$, where P is a polygonal identifier (or an identifier of some other areal unit) that replaces U and V. Thus, the geographic information in the masked data is reduced in dimensionality from two columns (U, V) to one column (P). Point aggregation, on the other hand, retains the original dimensionality by mapping each row of (U, V) to a point.

7.2.3 Affine Transformations

A second, relatively simple masking method, considered by Aldrich and Krautheim and Leitner and Curtis, is to move all locations of health events deterministically to new locations via a translation, scale change, or rotation of the underlying two-dimensional coordinate system.[17,18] Such operations, individually or in any combination, are known as *affine transformations*. A simple (rigid) translation mask yields the data matrix

$$M = [U + \Delta u \cdot e, V + \Delta v \cdot e, W, Z]$$

where Δu and Δv are fixed increments describing the shift in the x and y directions, respectively, and e is an n-by-1 vector of ones. A scale change occurs by multiplying each coordinate of each event by a scalar γ, that is,

$$M = [\gamma U, \gamma V, W, Z].$$

Finally, a rotation is obtained by evaluating

$$M = \left[(U,V) \begin{bmatrix} \cos\theta & -\sin\theta \\ \sin\theta & \cos\theta \end{bmatrix}, W, Z \right],$$

where θ is a fixed angle of rotation. Actually, this form of rotation uses the origin of the coordinate system as the pivot point around which events are rotated. To rotate about an arbitrary location requires that the events be translated, prior to rotation, by the displacement between the chosen pivot point and the origin of the coordinate system. Obviously, all three operations of translation, scaling, and rotation can be combined to increase the level of masking beyond that which obtains for any operation individually.

Elements of randomness can be incorporated easily into an affine transformation, if desired. For example, a stochastic translation mask could be implemented by taking Δu and Δv to be independent uniform random variables on the interval $(-\delta, \delta)$ for some $\delta > 0$; a stochastic rotation mask would result from taking θ to be a uniform random variable on the interval $(0, 2\pi)$.

Whether deterministic or stochastic, an affine transformation preserves exactly the relative locations and orientations of events.

7.2.4 RANDOM SPATIAL PERTURBATION

A third general technique for geographic masking is *random spatial perturbation*, which consists of displacing each event by a randomly determined amount in a randomly determined direction relative to its original location.[18,19] We can represent this mask as

$$M = [U + C, V + D, W, Z]$$

where the components of C and D are random variables. The difference between this approach and that of a stochastic affine transformation is that the random amount and direction of displacement are allowed to vary among events. Thus, random perturbation does not preserve exactly the relative locations and orientations of events.

Typically, the event-specific displacements will be taken to be independent and identically distributed random variables, but this is not necessary; in fact, for some purposes it may be undesirable. For example, when the population density is highly variable over the region of interest, it may be advisable to displace events in subregions of relatively low population density by larger (on average) amounts than events in subregions of high density to more nearly equalize the risk of disclosure across individuals. Cassa et al. described such a mask and showed, through a simulation with generated spatial data of emergency room visits, that spatial clusters in the original data could still be discovered using the SATScan algorithm after implementation of such a mask.[14] There may also be circumstances for which one would like displacements corresponding to nearby events to be positively correlated, such as when one desires the nearest-neighbor distances among events to be relatively unchanged by the perturbation.

A particular distribution or family of distributions must be chosen for the random displacements. Two useful distributional families for this purpose are the bivariate uniform and bivariate normal distributions. Each has its relative advantages. The bivariate uniform, for example, can easily accommodate irregularly shaped regions (because of the presence of coastlines, etc.) within which the event must lie after perturbation, and its displacements are bounded above by the distribution's range parameter. In contrast, the normal distribution cannot easily accommodate irregular regions, and its displacements are unbounded. However, imposing correlation between displacements is much more straightforward with the normal distribution than with the uniform distribution.

7.2.5 NEAREST-NEIGHBOR INFORMATION

Frequently, the main objective of a user of geographic health data is to investigate whether health events have occurred in spatial clusters. Many tests for clustering based on point-level data exist, of which most are functions of only the nearest-neighbor information in the data. Thus, for these situations it may be sufficient to provide the user with merely the desired nearest-neighbor information. Some clustering statistics (e.g., the Clark-Evans statistic) utilize distances to the nearest neighbor only, others use distances to the two or three nearest neighbors, and still others (e.g., the Cuzick-Edwards statistic) require knowledge of which type of event — a case or a control — is the nearest neighbor of each event. Local tests for clustering, which permit the user to determine not only whether but also where clustering has occurred, require some information on the locations of the events. This type of information could be given in aggregated form; that is, the subregion in which each event lies could be included with the nearest-neighbor distance, or the midpoint of the chord connecting an event to its nearest neighbor could be used to provide the necessary positional information.

7.2.6 ATTRIBUTE PERTURBATION

In some situations, the attribute information in Z is of such fine detail and is so readily available to users from a source independent of the data custodian that its release together with that of the geographically masked health information would increase the risk of a breach to an unacceptable level. These situations call for a mask not only of (U, V) but also of Z. Rushton et al. described a scenario in which such a mask is required.[11] In this scenario, the custodian of the geographic health data (a state health agency) lacks the expertise to perform appropriate spatial epidemiologic analyses of them. Therefore, the custodian solicits the assistance of a user (university researchers) for this purpose, in particular to investigate possible relationships between environmental contamination and health outcomes in a particular county. The user has the required expertise and has access, independently from the custodian, to detailed data on the environmental contamination at the residences of inhabitants of the county. Thus, in terms of our matrix notation, the user possesses $[U, V, Z]$; the custodian has $[U, V, W]$ and wants an analysis relating possible effects of Z on W. The obvious mode for this to occur would be for the custodian to provide the user with $[U, V, W]$, but this would clearly violate privacy laws or agreements under which the custodian collected the data. The next most obvious solution would be for the user to give $[U, V, Z]$ to the custodian and then have the custodian append W to it, strip it of (U, V) and then send $[W, Z]$ to the user for analysis. However, this would also amount to a breach of confidentiality because the user could easily recover (U, V) from the file of $[U, V, Z]$ in its possession and then match each row of $[W, Z]$ with the corresponding row of $[U, V, Z]$. The solution that Rushton et al. devised was for the user to provide the custodian with $[U, V, Z]$ but then have the custodian mask Z (e.g., by random perturbation) to obtain masked environmental contaminant values Z^* and then finally send $[W, Z^*]$ to the user for analysis. With the attribute so masked, the user cannot match health events with their corresponding spatial coordinates (and hence cannot match them to individual residences), yet enough accuracy can be retained in the attribute that the analysis of the contaminants' possible association with health outcomes may be only slightly affected. By weighing the benefits of a more powerful and accurate analysis against the risk and cost of possible disclosure, the custodian can determine the degree to which it will modify Z through masking.

7.2.7   IMPLEMENTATION

Most of the masking techniques reviewed can be implemented easily using standard GIS software. Some (e.g., affine transformations and random perturbation) can also be implemented using spreadsheets. For the remaining methods, purpose-specific programs must be written. Details of a random displacement algorithm within r distance with instructions for implementing it in the Microsoft program Excel are described in chapter 8.

7.3   EVALUATION OF APPROACHES

7.3.1   PRESERVING INFORMATION AND STRUCTURE

Every geographic mask results in some loss of information to the data user. However, some masks preserve more information than others, and some may preserve all the information that a user needs to answer a particular research question. Therefore, it is useful to evaluate masks regarding their information preservation characteristics. Relevant to this issue is the notion of a user-sufficient mask. A mask M is said to be user sufficient if the collection of quantities T needed by the user to address a question of interest is a function of the masked data; that is, if $T(X) = T(M(X))$. For example, if a user desires to investigate the possible existence of disease clusters using the Cuzick-Edwards test statistic, then any mask that preserves whether each case's nearest neighbor is a case or a control is user sufficient.

In practice, the needs of the data user cannot always be anticipated by the data custodian (or even by the data user), hence it is useful to evaluate the ability of a mask to preserve information along several dimensions, such as preservation of interpoint distances and orientations, distances to geographical features like highways or putative hazard sources, existence and location of clusters, and trends in the spatial density of events. For instance, translations preserve interpoint distances and orientations perfectly but do not preserve the locations of clusters. A thorough summary of the information preservation qualities of various geographic masks was provided by Armstrong et al. These authors concluded that random perturbation is the most robust all-purpose mask as it preserves reasonably accurate information along many dimensions.[12]

Most masks, unless they are user sufficient, will tend to obscure or reduce any spatial structure (e.g., clustering or trend) that exists in the original data. For example, a random perturbation mask tends to make a clustered pattern of health events less so,[20] and aggregation may obscure the clustering entirely.[21] On the other hand, random perturbation or aggregation of a completely random pattern of events typically does not yield a more clustered pattern. Thus, there is an asymmetry in the qualifications that should accompany the statistical inferences that a user of masked data makes from tests for spatial structure. More specifically, if a test statistic's magnitude is such that a structural attribute is deemed statistically significant, then no qualification is necessary. On the other hand, if the test indicates that a structural attribute is not statistically significant, then this inference should be qualified with a statement to the effect that masking could have prevented the detection of the attribute. It is possible for individual registries or other data custodians to conduct numerical studies of the effect of increasing perturbation on the detection of clusters or other types of structure with their data sets to determine a threshold level of perturbation at which there is an acceptable tradeoff between analytic power and disclosure risk.

7.3.2 PRESERVING LINKS TO OTHER GEOREFERENCED INFORMATION

A creative method for preserving privacy and protecting the confidentiality of individual data is for the holder of the individualized data to process the data to determine a relationship of value and to release information on the relationship. A "spider map" showing the place of diagnosis for a given cancer shows interesting spatial patterns of patient care. However, publishing such a map compromises assurances given to hospitals that the confidentiality of their records will be maintained. The relationship that the maker of such a map might be interested in showing is that people in some areas are diagnosed at longer distances than people living in other areas. Rushton et al., using density maps, showed the average distance of people living in an area to the location where their cancer was diagnosed.[22] In a second example, Olson et al. investigated the degree to which knowledge of the interpoint distances among patient locations could be used to detect disease clusters in a real-time syndromic surveillance system.[23] In an earlier article, Olson et al. developed a statistic that compared the expected proportion of distance values with the actual proportions using a nonparametric comparison based on the covariance matrix.[24] Using simulated disease outbreaks, they determined the sensitivity of the statistic to detect outbreaks of different sizes at different locations in the hospital service area. They concluded that the approach is powerful for detecting quite small outbreaks in both time and space.

7.3.3 PRESERVING CONFIDENTIALITY

It is also useful to evaluate geographic masks regarding how well they preserve confidentiality. For this purpose, several measures of confidentiality preservation or its complement, disclosure risk, have been proposed. Two of the most broadly useful measures are the area of a confidence region (of specified coverage probability) for the true location of an arbitrary health event, which is considered in further detail in the next section, and Spruill's measure,[25] defined in a spatial context as the proportion of records in the masked data matrix M with masked locations that are geographically closer to their corresponding true locations in X than to any other locations in X. Other useful measures include vulnerability to local geographic knowledge (i.e., how easily the mask can be decoded by constraints imposed by such features as rivers, lakes, topography, rectilinear road systems, etc.) and the minimum number of health events that, were the data user to link them to their obvious identifiers, would compromise the entire data set. Translation and the other affine transformations have a high disclosure risk with respect to these last two criteria; if the data were merely translated, then knowledge of local geographic features may allow the translated map to be easily "snapped back" to its original position. Similarly, the linkage of a single record to its obvious identifiers would permit a data user, on determining the true address (and hence the geographic coordinates) of that event, to reestablish the original coordinates (and hence the addresses) of every event. Armstrong et al.

evaluated various geographic masks with respect to these and other measures; they concluded that aggregation and nearest-neighbor masks have the lowest disclosure risk, followed by random perturbation, with affine transformation far behind.[12] It is not surprising, in light of the trade-off between information preservation and confidentiality preservation, that this order is the reverse of the order of masks with respect to information preservation we listed.

7.3.4 MASK METADATA AND MULTIPLE MASKS

Two important practical issues in geographic masking that have received attention only recently are mask metadata and multiple masks. *Mask metadata* refers to specific information about the mask that was applied to the data, for example, which type of mask was used (e.g., an affine transformation or random spatial perturbation) and which values were used for various parameters of the mask. The release of mask metadata to accompany the masked data assists users by allowing them, in principle, to determine how definitive the conclusions of their spatial analysis are or even whether conducting such an analysis is worthwhile. For example, suppose that the custodian randomly perturbs the locations of disease cases, with perturbations sampled randomly from a uniform distribution with radius 1 kilometer. Disclosing this information to data users can help them to determine whether any disease clusters identified by the statistical analysis are statistically significant. But, such a disclosure may also help a nefarious user intent on breaching confidentiality by eliminating from consideration as possible cases all individuals who reside outside circles of radius 1 kilometer centered on masked locations. Thus, the custodian must carefully consider the potential effects on confidentiality of the type and specificity of information disclosed in any mask metadata release.

The second issue, multiple masks, is another that a data custodian must consider carefully. This issue arises naturally because, as noted, the type and degree of geographic masking applied to the data affects the kinds of spatial analyses that may be performed as well as the strength of conclusions that can be drawn from the analyses. Because the data may be requested for the purpose of addressing a range of different research goals over time, by perhaps many users, it may be necessary for the custodian to release several masked versions of the data. A potential consequence of releasing multiple masked versions of the same data set is that a nefarious user or colluding users might be able to combine information from different releases to compromise confidentiality, even when each masked release by itself sufficiently preserves it.

Zimmerman and Pavlik quantified the extent to which confidentiality can be affected by the disclosure of mask metadata and multiple masked releases.[26] Here, we present two scenarios they considered. Suppose that the custodian releases m masked versions of the data, each a spatial perturbation mask, with perturbations randomly sampled from a bivariate normal distribution with mean vector 0 and covariance matrix $\sigma^2 I$. Suppose further that the specifics of the mask, including the variance parameter σ^2, are disclosed to users. Then, it can be shown that, for $0 < \alpha < 1$, the $100(1 - \alpha)\%$ confidence region for an arbitrary true location is a circle of radius $\sqrt{[(\sigma^2/m)\chi^2(2, \alpha)]}$ centered at the corresponding masked location, where

$\chi^2(2, \alpha)$ is the $100(1 - \alpha)$th percentile of a χ^2 distribution with two degrees of freedom. Thus, the confidence region's area is $\pi\sigma^2\chi^2(2, \alpha)/m$, from which the effect of multiple masked releases is revealed. That is, the level of confidentiality, as measured by the area of the confidence region, decreases at the rate of $1/m$ as the number m of masked releases increases. The expression for the confidence region's area can also provide guidance to the custodian; if, for instance, a policy existed on the minimal allowable area of a 95% confidence region for an arbitrary true location, then the expression could be used to solve for the largest value of m (for a given σ^2) or the smallest value of σ^2 (for given m) that would keep the custodian in compliance with the policy.

Now, consider a scenario similar to that just described but the value of σ^2 is not disclosed to users. Then, provided that there are at least two releases, a $100(1 - \alpha)\%$ confidence region for an arbitrary true location is a circle of radius $\sqrt{\{2s^2F[2,2n(m - 1), \alpha]/(m - 1)\}}$ centered at the corresponding masked location, where s^2 is the pooled (across cases) and averaged (across the two dimensions) sample variance of the displacements, and $F[2,2n(m - 1), \alpha]$ is the $100(1 - \alpha)$th percentile of an F distribution with 2 and $2n(m - 1)$ degrees of freedom. The expected area of this region is given by $2\pi\sigma^2F[2,2n(m - 1), \alpha]/m$. The ratio of the expected areas of the confidence regions, that is, $\chi^2(2, \alpha)/2F[2,2n(m - 1), \alpha]$, can be interpreted as a measure of the degradation in confidentiality because of disclosure of the perturbation variance σ^2; the smaller the ratio is, the greater the degradation will be. Based on the values of this ratio for various values of n, m, and α, Zimmerman and Pavlik (2006) showed that the disclosure of σ^2 typically results in a confidentiality degradation of 5%–20%, with a smaller effect as n and m increase.[26] This is not surprising in light of the fact that multiple releases of the masked data themselves can be used to construct an ever more precise estimate of σ^2 as n and m increase.

7.4 CONCLUSIONS

In this chapter, we summarized the key methods developed to mask individual-level information to protect confidentiality. These methods vary considerably in the amount of difficulty required to defeat them as well as in their ability to support particular types of analyses. Given the problems of protecting privacy by using geographic masks, we conclude by asking the following question: Are there alternatives to masking that protect privacy? There are a number of directions these alternatives follow.

Boulos et al. proposed the use of software agents that can perform spatial analyses on individually identifiable data and output results in which no individual identities are revealed or could be revealed by associating the results with other available information.[27] To implement this idea, they envisioned a computer firewall constructed to permit the request for access to the analysis knowing that the software used does not permit the protected data to be returned to the requestor.

A software agent mediates between the needs of a user and the need to protect the confidentiality of information. Users submit requests for an analysis to an agent, which accesses required information, performs an analysis, and releases a result, subject to confidentiality restrictions. It is even possible to have an agent create either a summary graph or map or generate one as a realization of a stochastic process.

Care must be taken, however, to prevent agents from releasing multiple results that could be integrated with other information or results to yield unacceptable levels of disclosure risk. Moreover, any map produced as a result of a stochastic process would yield a number of false positives, causing possible problems to individuals who are falsely identified.

A final approach is to support the development and use of protected enclaves. In such environments, users are required to sign statements that proscribe the use and release of confidential information outside the enclave. Typically, analyses of unmasked data are performed within the enclave, and only summary results are allowed to leave the protected environment. Enforcement of confidentiality agreements is left to legal (prosecution) and professional (censure) remedies. Enclaves also have an effect of reducing access to information because physical travel is typically required.

REFERENCES

1. Armstrong, M. P. Geographic information technologies and their potentially erosive effects on personal privacy. *Studies in the Social Sciences,* 27, 19–28, 2002.
2. Armstrong, M. P.; Ruggles, A. J. Geographic information technologies and personal privacy. *Cartographica,* 40, 63–73, 2005.
3. Curry, M. R. *Digital Places: Living with Geographic Technologies.* Routledge, New York, NY, 1997.
4. Matthews, S. A. *GIS and Privacy* (GIS Resource Document 03-51). February 2003. Population Research Institute, Pennsylvania State University.
5. Monmonier, M. S. *Spying with Maps: Surveillance Technologies and the Future of Privacy.* University of Chicago Press, Chicago, IL, 2002.
6. Pickles, J. *Ground Truth: The Social Implications of Geographic Information Systems.* Guilford, New York, NY, 1995.
7. Curry, M. R. Rethinking privacy in a geocoded world. In *Geographical Information Systems*, Longley, P. A.; Goodchild, M. F.; Maguire, D. J.; Rhind, D. W., Eds. Wiley, New York, 1999, Vol. 2, p. 757–766.
8. VanWey, L. K.; Rindfuss, R. R.; Gutmann, M. P.; Entwisle, B.; Balk, D. L. Confidentiality and spatially explicit data: concerns and challenges. *Proceedings of the National Academy of Sciences,* 102, 15337–15342, 2005.
9. Brownstein, J. S.; Cassa, C. A.; Kohane, I. S.; Mandl, K. D. An unsupervised classification method for inferring original case locations from low-resolution disease maps. *International Journal of Health Geographics*, 5, 56, 2006.
10. Brownstein, J. S.; Cassa, C. A.; Mandl, K. D. No place to hide — reverse identification of patients from published maps. *New England Journal of Medicine,* 355, 1741–1742, 2006.
11. Rushton, G.; Armstrong, M. P.; Gittler, J.; Greene, B. R.; Pavlik, C. E.; West, M. M.; Zimmerman, D. L. Geocoding in cancer research: a review. *American Journal of Preventive Medicine,* 30, S16–S24, 2006.
12. Armstrong, M. P.; Rushton, G.; Zimmerman, D. L. Geographically masking health data to preserve confidentiality. *Statistics in Medicine,* 18, 497–525, 1999.
13. Wartell, J.; McEwen, J. T. Privacy in the information age: a guide for sharing crime maps and spatial data. Institute for Law and Justice, NCJ 188739, 2001.
14. Cassa, C. A.; Grannis, S. J.; Overhage, J. M.; Mandl, K. D. A context-sensitive approach to anonymizing spatial surveillance data: impact on outbreak detection. *Journal of the American Medical Informatics Association,* 13, 160–165, 2006.

15. Duncan, G. T.; Pearson, R. W. Enhancing access to microdata while protecting confidentiality: prospects for the future. *Statistical Science,* 6, 219–231, 1991.

16. Daskin, M. S. *Network and Discrete Location: Models, Algorithms, and Applications.* Wiley, New York, NY, 1995.

17. Aldrich, T. E.; Krautheim, K. R. Protecting confidentiality in small area studies. In *CDC Symposium on Statistical Methods: Small Area Statistics in Public Health,* Atlanta, GA, 1995.

18. Leitner, M.; Curtis, A. Cartographic guidelines for geographically masking the locations of confidential point data. *Cartographic Perspectives,* 49, 22–39, 2004.

19. Kwan, M. P.; Casas, I.; Schmitz, B. C. Protection of geoprivacy and accuracy of spatial information: how effective are geographical masks. *Cartographica,* 39, 15–28, 2004.

20. Cox, D. R.; Isham, V. *Point Processes.* Chapman and Hall, London, 1980.

21. Olson, K. L.; Grannis, S. J.; Mandl, K. D. Privacy protection versus cluster detection in spatial epidemiology. *American Journal of Public Health,* 96, 2002–2008, 2006.

22. Rushton, G.; Peleg, I.; Banerjee, A.; Smith, G.; West, M. Analyzing geographic patterns of disease incidence: rates of late-stage colorectal cancer in Iowa. *Journal of Medical Systems,* 28, 223–236, 2004.

23. Olson, K. L.; Bonetti, M.; Pagano, M.; Mandl, K. D. Real time spatial cluster detection using interpoint distances among precise patient locations. *BMC Medical Informatics and Decision Making,* 5, 19, 2005.

24. Olson, K. L.; Bonetti, M.; Pagano, M.; Mandl, K. A population-adjusted stable geospatial baseline for outbreak detection in syndromic surveillance. *Morbidity and Mortality Weekly Report, Syndromic Surveillance Reports,* 53 (Suppl), 256, Sept. 24, 2004.

25. Spruill, N. L. The confidentiality and analytic usefulness of masked business microdata. *Proceedings of the Section on Survey Research Methods,* 602–607, 1983.

26. Zimmerman, D. L.; Pavlik, C. Quantifying the effects of mask metadata disclosure and multiple releases on the confidentiality of geographically masked health data. *Geographical Analysis* (in press).

27. Kamel Boulos, M. N.; Cai, Q.; Padget, J. A.; Rushton, G. Using software agents to preserve individual health data confidentiality in micro-scale geographical analyses. *Journal of Biomedical Informatics,* 39, 160–170, 2006.

8 Preserving Privacy
Deidentifying Data
by Applying a Random
Perturbation Spatial Mask

Zunqiu Chen, Gerard Rushton, and Geoffrey Smith

CONTENTS

8.1 INTRODUCTION

This chapter describes implementation steps for one of the methods for geographically masking locations that was discussed in reference [1] (p. 504) and called *random perturbation*. It also describes an implementation program in Microsoft Excel® for applying this method to a file of coordinates of locations. The input for this program is a set of coordinates and a selected parameter value for implementing the mask in miles, kilometers, meters, or feet, depending on your measurement unit. The output is the displaced coordinates of the set in longitude and latitude decimal degrees. This program can be downloaded from the Web site given.

We show how to mask a set of locations defined by longitude and latitude in decimal degrees. All locations will be displaced from their true locations using a random function that places each point at any equally likely location within r units of its true location. The unit can be miles, kilometers, meters, or feet. In the demonstration, we show the process and result in miles, although we provide formulae to allow the conversion to kilometers, meters, or feet into longitude and latitude in decimal degrees if the unit is in kilometers, meters, or feet.

8.2 PURPOSE

The purpose is to determine the longitude and latitude of "masked" points that have displaced values within a selected r miles maximum distance (set by the user) such that all locations within the circle are equally likely to be selected as the masked location for the true location in the center (Figure 8.1).

8.2.1 TRUE LOCATION

We begin with a given true location in longitude, latitude decimal coordinates. For example, we use the original location of a point with longitude = −91.3431 (OldLong) and latitude = 40.83927 (OldLat).

8.2.2 UNIFORMLY DISTRIBUTED RANDOM NUMBERS

First, generate two uniformly distributed random numbers within a range of $2r$ miles (Figure 8.2).

$$v_1 \sim U(-r,r)$$
$$v_2 \sim U(-r,r) \tag{8.1}$$

where v_1 is a uniformly distributed random number between $-r$ and $+ r \sim U(-r, r)$, where v_2 is a uniformly distributed random number between $-r$ and $+ r \sim U(-r, r)$, r is the radius of the circle of the mask in the given units-miles.

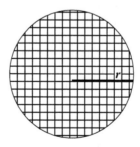

FIGURE 8.1 Spatial extent of the mask for the true location in the center (each square in the circle is equally likely to be selected by the masking algorithm).

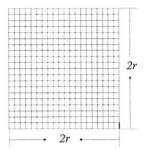

FIGURE 8.2 The extent of the area for two uniformly distributed random numbers.

8.2.3 ENSURE THE POINT IS CENTERED

Second, to ensure that the point is within a circle centered on the point, set up a condition for this pair of random numbers as follows:

$$v_1^2 + v_2^2 \leq r^2 \tag{8.2}$$

where v_1 is a uniformly distributed random number between $-r$ and $+r$ $\sim U(-r, r)$, where v_2 is a uniformly distributed random number between $-r$ and $+r$ $\sim U(-r, r)$, and r is the radius of the circle of the mask in the given units-miles.

Therefore, all generated points occur within the circle area (Figure 8.3).

Each point geocoded by this process has an equal likelihood of existing within a circle of radius r centered on the original location of the point to be masked. For example, take the original location of the point with longitude = −91.3431 and latitude = 40.83927 and reassign the coordinates of this point with $X = 0$ and $Y = 0$. Then, set the maximum distance r as 2.5 miles. Let those v_1 and v_2 satisfy the condition in Equation 8.2. The output based on this step shows 1000 simulated points for the true location in the center of Figure 8.4.

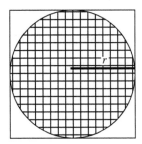

FIGURE 8.3 The extent of the circle area for the masked point locations.

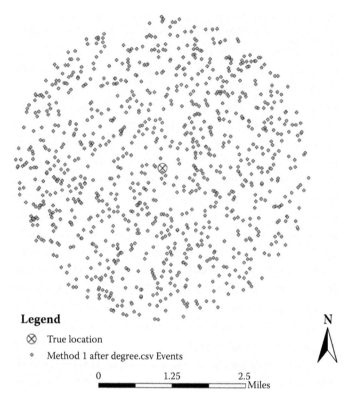

Legend

⊗   True location

◇   Method 1 after degree.csv Events

```
0                    1.25                    2.5
                                                Miles
```

FIGURE 8.4 Locations of 1000 simulated points with $r = 2.5$ miles.

8.3 CONVERT DISPLACEMENT DISTANCES

Third, the displacement distances v_1 and v_2 in the given units need to be converted into new coordinates of location (latitude and longitude) because the original location is in longitude and latitude decimal coordinates. We compute the change in latitude (see section 8.6.1) and the change in longitude (see section 8.6.2) using the formulae presented next.

8.3.1 CONVERSION OF DISPLACEMENT IN GIVEN UNITS TO LATITUDE DEGREES

For displacement in miles, the change is

$$\Delta \text{ Degree } Y = \frac{v_2}{69.17} \qquad (1 \text{ degree latitude} = 69.17 \text{ miles}) \qquad (8.3)$$

For displacement in kilometers,

$$\Delta \text{ Degree } Y = \frac{v_2}{69.17 \times 1.609} \quad (1 \text{ degree latitude} = 69.17 \times 1.609 \text{ kilometers}) \quad (8.4)$$

For displacement in meters,

$$\Delta \text{ Degree } Y = \frac{v_2}{69.17 \times 1609} \quad (1 \text{ degree latitude} = 69.17 \times 1609 \text{ meters}) \quad (8.5)$$

For displacement in feet,

$$\Delta \text{ Degree } Y = \frac{v_2}{69.17 \times 5280} \quad (1 \text{ degree latitude} = 69.17 \times 5280 \text{ feet}) \quad (8.6)$$

8.3.2 CONVERSION OF DISPLACEMENT IN GIVEN UNITS TO LONGITUDE DEGREES

To convert distance in given units to longitude degrees, we need to compensate for the fact that the east-west distance direction along a parallel (a line of latitude) between two meridians (lines of longitude) one degree apart becomes progressively less toward the pole; a scalar factor that depends on the specific latitude of the address must be used in the formula for computing the mask. A more detailed explanation of this phenomenon can be found in Kirvan[2] and Robinson et al.[3] To calculate the length of a degree of longitude one can multiply the cosine of the latitude by 69.17 miles (the length of a degree at the equator).[3] An alternative distance calculator can be found on the website of the National Geospatial-Intelligence Agency (http://pollux.nss. nima.mil/calc/degree.html). Select "Nautical Calculators," then select "distance" to find a page that "allows calculation of one degree of latitude and longitude. Lengths are calculated in nautical miles, statute miles, feet, and meters."

For displacement in miles where OldLat is the latitude of the original point, the change is

$$\Delta \text{ Degree } X = \frac{v_1}{69.17} \div \cos\left(\frac{\text{OldLat}}{180} \times \pi\right) \quad (8.7)$$

For displacement in kilometers,

$$\Delta \text{ Degree } X = \frac{v_1}{69.17 \times 1.069} \div \cos\left(\frac{\text{OldLat}}{180} \times \pi\right) \quad (8.8)$$

For displacement in meters,

$$\Delta \text{ Degree } X = \frac{v_1}{69.17 \times 1069} \div \cos\left(\frac{\text{OldLat}}{180} \times \pi\right) \tag{8.9}$$

For displacement in feet,

$$\Delta \text{ Degree } X = \frac{v_1}{69.17 \times 5280} \div \cos\left(\frac{\text{OldLat}}{180} \times \pi\right) \tag{8.10}$$

8.4 CALCULATE LATITUDE OF MASKED POINT

Fourth, to calculate the new latitude of the masked point, add the Y displacement (Degree Y) to the old latitude:

$$\text{NewLat } Y = \text{OldLat} + \Delta \text{ Degree } Y$$

OldLat: the latitude of the original point

$$\tag{8.11}$$

To calculate the new longitude of the masked point, add the X displacement (DegreeX) to the old longitude:

$$\text{NewLong } X = \text{OldLong} + \Delta \text{ Degree } X$$

OldLong : the longitude of the original point

$$\tag{8.12}$$

These steps are to generate random points with equal likelihood within a circle of radius r centered on the original location of the point to be masked in longitude and latitude coordinates (independent of the projection). For example, we still use the original location of a point with longitude = −91.3431 (OldLong) and latitude = 40.83927 (OldLat). Then, set the maximum distance as 2.5 miles. The output, in Figure 8.5, shows an elliptical shape of 1000 simulated random points for the true location before they are projected to a suitable coordinate system.

8.5 THE PROJECTED MAP

Finally, after using a suitable projection (in this case, 1983_UTM_Zone_15N for the State of Iowa using ArcGIS® software) for the output, Figure 8.6 shows the projected map.

The output from Figure 8.6 fulfills the purpose of generating random points with equal likelihood within a circle of radius r centered on the original location of the point.

To use this Mask Program download from http://www.uiowa.edu/~gishlth

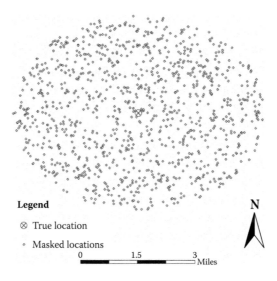

FIGURE 8.5 Locations of 1000 simulated points with $r = 2.5$ miles (independent of the projection).

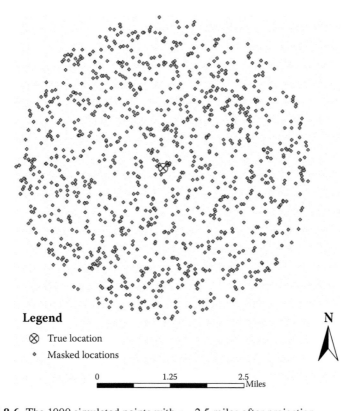

FIGURE 8.6 The 1000 simulated points with $r = 2.5$ miles after projection.

REFERENCES

1. Armstrong, M. P.; Rushton, G.; Zimmerman, D. L. Geographically masking health data to preserve confidentiality. *Statistics in Medicine* 1999, 18, 497–525.
2. Kirvan, A. P. Latitude/longitude, NCGIA core curriculum in GIScience. 1997. http://www.ncgia.ucsb.edu/giscc/units/u014/u014.html (accessed July 21, 2007).
3. Robinson, A. R.; Morrison, J. L.; Muehrcke, P. C.; Guptill, S. C. *Elements of Cartography*, Wiley, New York, 1995.

9 Spatial Statistical Analysis of Point- and Area-Referenced Public Health Data

Lance A. Waller

CONTENTS

9.1 INTRODUCTION

Once we have geocoded health-related data, what sort of questions can we answer? A wide variety of spatial analytic tools are available addressing different substantive questions of interest, so it is important to realize that the choice of analytic tool often predisposes the sort of question addressed. As a result, care must be taken in choosing an analytic approach that is appropriate to the question of interest and the available data. In the sections in this chapter, we provide an overview of common questions asked of georeferenced health data and associated statistical methods for answering those questions.

The first distinction often used to classify spatial analytic methods is based on the structure of the underlying geocoded data. In this review, we consider two primary data classes: data geocoded to point locations and data geocoded to areal units subdividing the region of interest. The distinction not only may be based on whether the geocoding process is capable of generating point locations from residential addresses but also may reflect confidentiality restrictions prohibiting release of geographic data at the point level.

Although accurate point data are often the goal of geocoding, many factors influence the spatial resolution desired in a particular analysis. First, it is important to consider whether a point location represents the location appropriate for the study at hand. As an example, Maxcy[1] illustrated stark differences between patterns observed in residential versus occupational point locations in an outbreak of endemic typhus in the 1920s, with occupational locations of cases revealing clearer clues to the etiology of the disease.[2] In addition, census data aggregated to census regions (e.g., blocks, block groups, or tracts) often provide important, albeit aggregate, background information on the population at risk. Finally, we may wish to model areal counts of incidence rather than the points themselves simply because of the wider availability of methods and software for modeling regional counts rather than spatial point patterns.

Within these two classes of data, there is a variety of questions of interest. For point data, we review methods addressing variants of the question: Does the observed pattern of point locations appear random, or do events appear to be clustered? For areal count data, we consider variations of the question: What associations do we observe between the observed counts and covariate values measured in the same regions?

The sections provide an overview of several specific statistical approaches for both point- and area-referenced data. More thorough descriptions of methods and additional examples appear in texts focusing on the applied[3,4] and more theoretical[5–7] levels of spatial statistical analysis.

9.2 ANALYZING POINT LOCATION DATA

Besag and Newell[8] distinguished between statistical approaches to identify individual clusters from approaches to identify clustering. A *cluster* refers to a set of observations seeming anomalous to the rest of the observed pattern; while *clustering* refers to a general pattern among all observations wherein observations tend to occur near other observations. The question of identifying individual clusters or general patterns of clustering within a set of point locations is deceptively simple to ask but complicated to answer quantitatively. Generally, tests to detect clusters seek to identify the set of observations that in some sense appear to be arranged in a pattern least consistent with the remaining observations; that is, these observations represent the most likely cluster. We note that even a truly random pattern will undoubtedly contain some apparent clusters; for example, independent tosses of a fair coin will result in some runs of consecutive heads. Therefore, it is important to assign some sort of measure of statistical significance to the most likely cluster representing how unusual such a collection would be by chance (i.e., under a null hypothesis of no clustering). In contrast, tests of clustering often represent single summary measures of relatedness among observed locations, often averaging some quantified measure of association between each observed location and its neighbors. We explore three approaches to these questions: The first visually represents spatial variation in the average number of events per unit area, the second identifies and evaluates the most likely cluster within the observed data, and the third assesses the degree of clustering by examining patterns among each event's nearest neighboring events.

Once we have a statistic measuring the most likely cluster or the overall degree of clustering, we next need to compare its observed value to the distribution of such a summary under a null hypothesis of no clustering. To assess statistical significance, we need to build from some basic probability components of models of random spatial point processes. We then base statistical inference on a general simulation-based tool for statistical inference: the Monte Carlo hypothesis test.

More specifically, the discussion implies the existence of some model of the absence of clustering, that is, a model of a truly random pattern of points. Mathematically, such a model is supplied by a homogeneous spatial Poisson process, also known as *complete spatial randomness* (CSR).[4,5,9] For our purposes, the defining features of CSR are two-fold: The total number of events observed follows a Poisson distribution, and given the total number observed, the event locations are uniformly distributed across the study area. Note that the term *uniformly* does not mean equally spaced but rather that each event is equally likely to occur at any possible point in the study area regardless of the locations of other events. The expected number of events is defined by the *intensity* of the process, that is, the average number of events per unit area. Under the properties of a Poisson point process, not only does the total number of events observed under CSR follow a Poisson distribution with mean equal to the intensity multiplied by the geometric area of the study region, but also the number of events observed in any subregion follows a Poisson distribution with mean defined by the product of the intensity and the area of the subregion. This feature provides a mathematical connection between point and areal data sets, motivating some of the statistical approaches for areal data considered in the next section.

In health studies, we often wish to extend the CSR model to account for spatially varying populations at risk. For instance, if the study area includes both towns and rural areas, a collection of five cases may be suspicious in a rural area with low population density but commonplace in a more densely populated setting with more individuals at risk. As a result, we may wish to make some allowance for the number of individuals at risk. We can accomplish this by allowing the intensity (number of events per unit area) to vary across the study region. This generalization, known as a *heterogeneous spatial Poisson process*, maintains many of the convenient properties mentioned, namely, the events still occur independently of one another and counts of events in subregions still follow Poisson distributions with means defined by the spatially varying intensity. However, events are more likely to occur in areas of high intensity and less likely to occur in areas of low intensity. Note that such a process will generate clusters of events in areas of high intensity, but these are clusters defined by known variations in the at-risk population. Most cluster investigations seek to focus attention on clustering above and beyond that expected simply caused by variations in the at-risk population.

In summary, the heterogeneous Poisson process provides a conceptual and mathematical basis for many tests to detect clusters or tests of clustering in point-referenced data. We review three types of tests to detect clusters based on these ideas, one based on estimates of the spatially varying intensity function, the next on a moving window defining local risks, and the third on nearest-neighbor classifications. All three tests assume a set of point locations for cases and a second set of point locations for noncases referred to as *controls*. The pattern of the controls represents the (heterogeneous) spatial intensity of the underlying population at risk, and we wish to compare the intensity of the cases to that of the controls. Any difference observed between the two intensities represents differences in the underlying point patterns and could identify potential clusters. For nearest neighbors, we investigate whether cases tend to be overrepresented among the nearest neighbors of other cases with respect to patterns expected if disease incidence is constant among individuals at risk.

To estimate the spatial intensity of a point process, we use a nonparametric method known as *kernel estimation*.[3,4,9] Conceptually, consider placing an identical lump of soft modeling clay at each observed case location. The lumps overlap for cases occurring near each other. If we consider the entire surface of modeling clay, then we have a spatially heterogeneous surface with peaks in areas with many events and valleys in areas with few events. The intensity for controls may be constructed in a similar manner. In general, let us define $\lambda(s)$ to be the intensity function at location s within the study region, and let $s_1, s_2, ..., s_n$ represent n observed point locations. We estimate $\lambda(s)$ by $\lambda_{kern}(s)$, defined by

$$\lambda_{kern}(s) = (1/b) * \sum kern[(s - s_i)/b]$$

where kern() is a kernel function representing our conceptual lump of clay, and b is the *bandwidth*, a measure of the spread of the kernel function.[9,10] The function kern() is peaked at the center and declining in a symmetric manner in all directions. The value $kern[(s - s_i)/b]$ is the height of the particular kernel centered at s_i with bandwidth b, evaluated at location s. Therefore, the kernel estimate is the sum of the heights at s of the kernels centered at each data location.

To illustrate this idea, consider the following case-control point data originally presented by Cuzick and Edwards[11] and representing the residential locations of 62 cases and 141 controls in North Humberside, England. Case locations represent residence locations for diagnoses of childhood leukemia or lymphoma in the period 1974–1986, and controls were randomly selected from residences from birth registrations between January 7 and July 7 for each year in the period 1974–1986. Locations represent centroids of the postal code of residence.

Figure 9.1 represents the data locations for cases and controls along with contours representing the estimated intensity functions for each pattern. We note immediately the spatial heterogeneity in the population at risk as evidenced by the nonuniform distribution of control locations. The intensity function contains a large peak near the south-central aggregation of cases and controls and another, smaller peak in the northeastern corner. No obvious differences in spatial pattern appear; rather, the spatial patterns of cases and controls appear similar.

In contrast to estimation and comparison of the respective intensity functions, the spatial scan statistic provides a more direct approach for identifying the most likely cluster (i.e., the most unusual set of cases). A rich body of scan statistic literature exists,[12] but it is the particular derivation and accompanying software implementation (SaTScan)[13] that is directly responsible for the large number of public health applications of spatial (and space-time) scan statistics. Scan statistics draw on a simple idea: Suppose we move a circular window across the study area and compare the ratio of cases to controls observed inside the window to that observed outside the window. If there is a local aggregation of cases, then we hope to identify it by capturing this aggregation within our window and noting a large difference between the case/control ratio inside the window compared to that outside the window. To capture different potential cluster sizes, we can consider a family of windows with radii ranging from the minimum distance between events to, say, one-half the area of the study region. In this setting, the most unusual collection of cases may be defined by the window containing the maximum case/control ratio. The degree to which this most likely cluster is unusual is measured by its observed value of the case/control ratio.

Now, some window will contain the most unusual collection even in the absence of clustering, so it is important to define an inferential structure for interpreting the

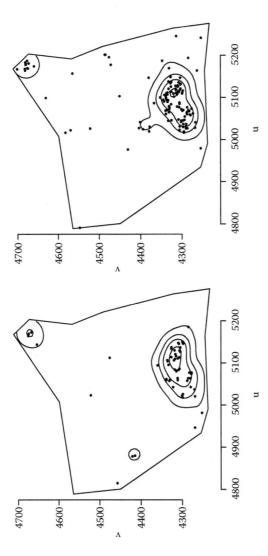

FIGURE 9.1 Spatial pattern of leukemia cases (left) and controls (right), 1974–1986, North Humberside, England. Contours represent kernel estimates of the spatial intensity of each pattern.

statistical significance of the observed value. Earlier window-based approaches such as the Geographic Analysis Machine[14] focus on assessing significance for each potential cluster compared to the expected number of cases at the same location, resulting in a separate test for each potential cluster and a statistical multiple-comparisons problem. Kulldorff,[13] on the other hand, recast the question of whether each local case/control ratio appears unusual for its location to the question of whether the observed maximum ratio appears unusual among the distribution of possible maximum ratios observed in the absence of clustering, regardless of where these maxima occur. A closed-form algebraic definition of this distribution is difficult to define analytically without restrictive assumptions, but Kulldorff noted that a simulation-based approach is fairly straightforward. Specifically, if we observe n_{case} cases and $n_{control}$ controls, under a null hypothesis of no clustering we would expect any random assignment of n_{case} cases among the n_{case} + $n_{control}$ locations to be equally likely, so we can compare the observed maximum case/control ratio across all window radii to the maximum observed under random assignment of the cases among the study locations. Such Monte Carlo tests are commonly used for clustering tests because simulation under the null hypothesis is simple even though analytic calculations are difficult.[9]

To illustrate the scan statistic approach, consider the North Humberside case-control data from Figure 9.1. Figure 9.2 shows two circles, each containing the maximum

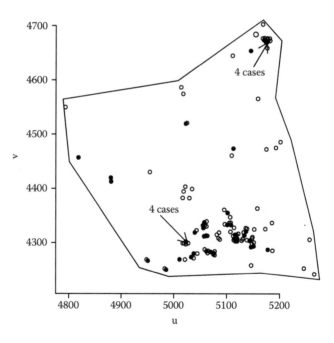

FIGURE 9.2 The most likely clusters in the North Humberside leukemia data based on the spatial scan statistic. Open circles represent control locations, filled circles represent case locations, and arrows indicate the locations of the two most unusual collections of cases (each containing 4 observed cases with 1.22 cases expected under the null hypothesis). Neither collection is statistically significant.

observed case/control ratio of 3.274, over a tripling of disease risk. However, the circles containing this observed value both contain only 4 cases in small geographic areas. Based on 999 random assignments of cases among the total set of locations, we obtain a (Monte Carlo) significance value of only 0.691 for each of the two clusters; that is, approximately 69% of the random permutations resulted in most likely clusters with higher local relative risks than that observed in the original data. This example illustrates that the most likely cluster is not necessarily a statistically unusual cluster of cases.

So far, the North Humberside data reveal little or no evidence of any local clusters, but what about clustering? Cuzick and Edwards[11] first introduced these data to illustrate a nearest-neighbor approach in which one examines the number of cases found within the m nearest neighbors of other cases. For each value of m, this number represents a summary across the entire data set indicating how likely one is to observe additional cases among the neighbors of other cases (i.e., a measure of clustering). Again using a Monte Carlo hypothesis test, we can assess statistical significance by comparing the observed nearest neighborhood case count to those resulting from randomly permuting the 62 cases among the 203 case-control locations. To illustrate the methodology, Figure 9.3 plots the observed number of cases among the 3, 5, 7, 9, 11, 13, and 15 nearest neighbors of each case, as well as a box plot of the simulated values based on 999 Monte Carlo simulations. The values for even numbers of nearest neighbors are comparable and are not shown so that a greater

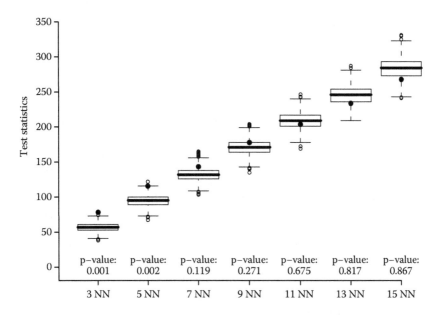

FIGURE 9.3 The filled circles represent the number of additional cases within the nearest neighbors of all cases in the North Humberside leukemia data. Box plots represent the distribution of additional cases within the nearest neighbors for 999 random permutations of 62 cases among the 203 total locations of cases and controls. The p values represent the proportion of values from the permuted data that generate more extreme numbers of cases among the nearest neighbors than those observed.

range of values may be illustrated. Significance levels (based on 999 random permutations) appear below each box plot and mirror the original analysis reported in Cuzick and Edwards.[11] We see statistically significant clustering of cases among the 3 and 5 nearest neighbors but not for larger numbers of nearest neighbors.

How do we reconcile the similar intensities in Figure 9.1, the nonsignificant most likely cluster in Figure 9.2, and the significant clustering demonstrated in Figure 9.3? Recall from the introduction that different methods assess different aspects of the spatial pattern of data, and we must interpret each result based on the type of evidence summarized by the method applied. Considering the tests involved, several features of the data become apparent. First, the scan statistic results in Figure 9.2 suggest that there does not appear to be a single collection of cases (at least captured by circular windows) comprising a cluster of events with pattern different from the rest of the study area. Second, the nearest-neighbor results in Figure 9.3 suggest there is some statistical evidence of cases occurring in collections of three to five nearest neighbors but not larger groups. In the North Humberside data, no single collection of cases presents strong evidence of a cluster, but our test of clustering identifies an overall pattern of relatively weak individual clusters occurring across the study area.

9.3 ANALYZING AREAL COUNT DATA

Confidentiality restrictions often limit the release and reporting of point data and in some instances (e.g., the U.S. Census) only aggregate values are available. Because such data are often used in public health studies to define characteristics of the population at risk, we next turn attention to analytic methods derived for aggregate counts. In most cases, the same underlying health questions drive investigations, but the data provide less spatial detail, and analytic methods must be adjusted accordingly.

To illustrate this, we begin with a generalization of the spatial scan statistic described for application to areal counts. For areal count data, we often replace the control pattern with census-based population counts for the subregions under study. The number at risk in each subregion defines the number of cases expected under a null hypothesis of no clusters. One can also use census demographics such as age to further refine the number expected within each region if disease risk varies by age or other individual-level characteristics. As with the point-based scan statistic, we again move circular windows of varying radii across the study area and compare the ratio of observed to expected numbers of cases inside the window to the same ratio outside the window. Each window location and radius defines a potential cluster, and as above, we seek to find the most unusual collection of cases, the "most likely cluster." In the area-based scan statistic, Kulldorff[13] included subregions within a potential cluster if the centroid of the subregion fell within the radius of the circular window. Extensions to other shapes of clusters are available,[15] but to date most applications use circular windows to detect clusters.

As with the point data approaches, establishing the statistical significance of the observed most likely cluster is important because, as before, some collection of cases will be least consistent with the null hypothesis, but it may not necessarily represent a statistically unusual aggregation. Monte Carlo simulation again plays a pivotal role because it is fairly straightforward to randomly assign cases to individuals at risk and obtain a sample of case patterns under a model of no clustering. By calculating the test statistic for each of these simulated data sets, we obtain a distribution of our test statistic under the null hypothesis.

To illustrate the scan statistic approach for areal count data, we consider a data set containing census tract counts for the period 1978–1982 of 592 leukemia deaths (the cases) among 1,057,673 people at risk in an eight-county region of upstate New York.[16,17] As with most real data sets, some compromises were necessary to include all available information. For example, not all cases could be geocoded with certainty to a single tract. Those cases with census tract of residence that could not be uniquely identified were assigned to the tracts possibly containing them, typically to one of a set of contiguous census tracts. In these instances, we assigned a fraction of a case corresponding to the fraction of the population at risk within the set of identified tracts. As a result, most tracts contain some fractional cases within their count.

Application of the spatial scan statistic to the New York leukemia data reveals the most likely cluster shown in Figure 9.4. Based on 999 random assignments of

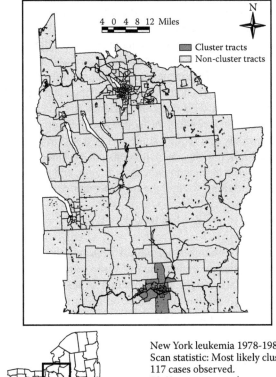

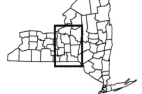

New York leukemia 1978-1982
Scan statistic: Most likely cluster
117 cases observed.
70.61 cases expected
Relative risk: 1.657
Monte Carlo p-value: 0.001

FIGURE 9.4 The dark gray tracts identify the most likely cluster in the New York leukemia data based on the spatial scan statistic.

592 cases among the population at risk, we find that only one of these simulated data sets generates a test statistic greater than that observed in the data, yielding a significance value of 0.001. This suggests that the most likely cluster represents a collection of cases unlikely to have arisen by chance and merits further investigation.

To further explore this pattern, we may wish to include additional risk factors to see if they help explain the observed patterns. The use of regression models provides a standard method for exploring linear relationships between a value of interest and a set of independent variables. In the spatial setting, both independent and dependent variables are matched by census region, and the usual statistical assumptions of independent errors may not hold, leading to the introduction of residual spatial autocorrelation. The literature contains many applications of adjustments to linear regression to account for spatially correlated errors,[18] but such models still maintain many assumptions, such as constant variance and normally distributed errors, that may not be met by areal counts of health events.

Waller and Gotway[9] provided a thorough exploration of modeling issues using the New York leukemia data, and we provide an overview here to highlight particular modeling strategies. For illustration, we follow Waller and Gotway[9] and consider two tract-specific covariates based on 1980 census data, namely, the percentage of residents aged 65 years or greater and the percentage of owner-occupied homes. In addition, we include a covariate summarizing proximity of the centroid of each tract to the nearest of 11 inactive hazardous waste sites listed as containing trichloroethylene (TCE) by the New York Department of Environmental Conservation.[19]

As mentioned, linear regression assumes that dependent variables follow a normal (Gaussian) distribution with constant variance and mean determined by the associated values of the independent variables. Areal counts, particularly for a rare disease, often vary widely and require some sort of transformation to approximate a normally distributed random variable with constant variance. If we define Y_i as the observed number of cases in region i, where $i = 1,\ldots, n$, and p_i as the resident population size for the same region,[9] we find the transformation

$$Z_i = \log(1000(Y_i + 1)/p_i)$$

to provide values approximating a normal distribution, with the exception of three large values corresponding to a collection of three census tracts in Syracuse, New York, with small population sizes and a fraction of a single observed case spread between them. Although we could consider omitting these observations, the fact that they represent large crude rates complicates the decision as they might well include important information regarding the spatial distribution of covariates and outcomes. Instead, we compensate for nonconstant variance in the transformed variables by using weighted least squares estimation, which assumes independence but not constant variance, instead of ordinary least squares estimation, which assumes both independence and constant variance. The impact of this decision is seen in Tables 9.1 and 9.2, showing the ordinary and weighted least squares results, respectively. The primary impact of allowing heterogeneous variances is the change in the effect associated with the proximity to the TCE sites, which becomes significant when we adjust for the increased variance observed in the three outliers.

TABLE 9.1

Ordinary Least Squares Estimates of Linear Regression Parameters for the New York Leukemia Data

Effect	Estimate	Standard Error	p Value
Intercept	−0.517	0.159	.001
Proximity to TCE site	0.049	0.035	.165
% age 65 years or older	3.951	0.606	< .001
% owner occupied	−0.560	0.170	.001

Source: Adapted from reference 9.

We note that both the ordinary least squares (Table 9.1) and the weighted least squares (Table 9.2) estimates assume independent error terms. We next consider incorporating a spatial correlation structure through a maximum likelihood estimation approach. Recall that maximum likelihood and least squares estimation approaches are equivalent for independent, symmetrically distributed error distributions, but only maximum likelihood extends to allow for correlated errors. Because of the heterogeneous subregion size illustrated in Figure 9.4, we choose a correlation structure with parameters defining a smooth distance decay in the correlation between tracts up to a distance of approximately 6.9 kilometers, beyond which we assume observations are independent.[9] Table 9.3 provides a summary of the impact of including spatially correlated errors on regression-based inference for the model. We see the impact of proximity to a TCE site increases slightly, and that the percentage of owner-occupied residences becomes nonsignificant, suggesting a spatial pattern in home ownership driving the association measured in Table 9.2.

Thus far, we have encountered the following complications to the basic linear regression model: nonnormality of the outcome, nonconstant variance, and nonindependence of error terms. Each was adjusted for in turn, but in some sense the

TABLE 9.2

Weighted Least Squares Estimates of Linear Regression Parameters for the New York Leukemia Data

Effect	Estimate	Standard Error	p Value
Intercept	−0.778	0.141	<.001
Proximity to TCE site	0.076	0.027	.006
% age 65 years or older	3.857	0.571	<.001
% owner occupied	−0.399	0.153	.010

Source: Adapted from reference 9.

TABLE 9.3

Weighted Maximum Likelihood Estimates of Linear Regression Parameters for the New York Leukemia Data, Accounting for Residual Spatial Autocorrelation

Effect	Estimate	Standard Error	p Value
Intercept	−0.916	0.165	< .001
Proximity to TCE site	0.096	0.032	.003
% age 65 years or older	3.576	0.592	< .001
% owner occupied	−0.229	0.176	.196

Source: Adapted from reference 9.

analysis is bound by these incremental steps, and the end result of all the adjustments may muddy relationships between variables on the original scale.

Another approach is to attempt to model the observed counts directly, using regression-type models for counts such as logistic or Poisson regression. Such models are members of the class of generalized linear models.[20] Such models are popular in the public health fields of biostatistics and epidemiology, but most applications assume independent observations. We quickly review such models and their extensions for spatially correlated error terms.

The basic structure of a generalized linear model involves a dependent variable Y_i assumed to follow some distribution such as normal (Gaussian) for continuous data or binomial or Poisson for count data. The expected (mean) value of the dependent variable is modeled as a function of independent variables through a function linking the expected outcome to a linear combination of covariates. For Poisson counts, it is typical to define a natural logarithm link resulting in the Poisson regression model

$$\log[E(Y_i)] = \beta_0 + \beta_1 x_1 + \cdots + \beta_q x_q$$

for q independent variables. This can also be expressed in terms of the number of cases expected E_i in each subregion as follows:

$$Y_i \sim \text{Poisson}[E_i \exp(\mu_i)],$$

where

$$\mu_i = \beta_0 + \beta_1 x_1 + \cdots + \beta_q x_q.$$

In this setting, the model parameters may be interpreted as the natural logarithm of the relative risk associated with a unit increase in the associated independent variable. That is, a unit increase in x_1 results in a multiplicative increase of $\exp(\beta_1)$

in the expected value of Y_i. The Poisson model has the attractive feature that if the underlying point locations for cases were assumed to follow a heterogeneous Poisson process as defined in the preceding section, we would expect the subregion counts to follow Poisson distributions.

Adding spatial correlation to generalized linear models is complicated by the fact that, for Poisson and binomial distributions, the mean and variance structures are interrelated, so modifying one necessarily modifies the other. The literature on statistical methods for disease mapping provides a useful extension to the Poisson regression model through the addition of subregion-specific random effects, that is, mean zero local adjustments to the intercept that, on average, do not add to the mean count but allow neighboring counts to be correlated.

More specifically, consider the following statistical model:

$$Y_i \sim \text{Poisson}[E_i \exp(\mu_i)],$$

where

$$\mu_i = \beta_0 + \beta_1 x_1 + \cdots + \beta_q x_q + \varphi_i,$$

and we assume the φ_i values have mean zero but are spatially correlated with one another. The addition of a parameter with specified distribution fits into a Bayesian statistical paradigm in which one defines prior distributions for model parameters, then updates these distributions based on the likelihood function defined by the observed data, resulting in a posterior distribution for each parameter.[6,9,21,22]

In the Bayesian setting, statistical inference is based on these posterior distributions. To complete a Bayesian specification for the model, we assume normal prior distributions with wide variances for the β_j parameters, indicating little prior precision. Such priors contain little information on the values of the parameters and allow the likelihood to identify their associated posterior distributions. For the φ_i parameters, we construct a more explicit set of prior distributions to induce the desired spatial correlation. The set of conditionally autoregressive prior distributions provides a convenient family for spatial modeling,[23,24] by which we define the conditional distribution for each φ_i conditional on the values of the other φ_k values where k is not equal to i. More explicitly, assume that

$$\varphi_i \mid \varphi_k \sim N[(\Sigma_k w_{ik} \varphi_k / \Sigma_k w_{ik}), 1/(\tau_\varphi^2 \Sigma_k w_{ik})]$$

so each φ_i is normally distributed around a weighted sum of the other φ_k values. Weights are typically defined by binary adjacencies (i.e., $w_{ik} = 1$ if subregions i and k are adjacent, 0 otherwise), but more general weights are also allowed. Note that the conditional variance around the weighted mean is a function of the sum of the weights. Besag[25] showed that such a set of conditional distributions defines a joint multivariate normal distribution with spatial correlation, precisely the effect we wish to include.

Prior to 1990, fitting Bayesian models involved complex integration or numerical approximations, but the advent of Markov chain Monte Carlo (MCMC) simulation-based approximations to these integrals now allows routine fitting of models such as the one outlined. MCMC algorithms begin with initial values for each model parameter, then update each value by simulating new values in such a manner that the set of simulated values converges to a random sample from the joint posterior distribution of all model parameters.

To illustrate this sort of model, we again consider the New York leukemia data set and fit the model using the WinBUGS software package,[26] which provides MCMC inference for such spatial models. Bayesian inference revolves around the posterior distribution for each parameter, so if we consider the same covariates as in our regression analysis, we wish to report the posterior median and a 95% credible set for each parameter (the range of values having 0.95 posterior probability of containing each parameter). Table 9.4 presents these posterior summaries. We note that the numeric values of the parameter estimates (the posterior medians) reflect log relative risks and are not directly comparable to those from the linear regressions. However, the effects are in the same directions, with positive values indicating factors increasing the expected number of cases and negative values indicating factors decreasing the expected counts. We note that the credible sets for percentage of residents with age ≥65 years or older and proximity to TCE sites both exclude zero, indicating strong posterior support for the impact of these variables on the outcome.

An advantage to a Bayesian approach based on MCMC methods is that we obtain a sample of values from the posterior distribution of any function of model parameters by simply keeping track of that function of parameters at each iteration of the MCMC algorithm. For example, if we are interested in the local standardized mortality ratio (SMR), defined as the ratio of the local fitted values predicted by the model and the expected counts in the absence of covariate values given the E_i values, we can calculate the fitted value based on each set of simulated values of model parameters and obtain a value of the SMR for each region. Taken across MCMC simulations, these values represent samples from the posterior distribution of each SMR. These allow us to map local estimates of SMRs to view areas with mortality higher or lower than expected. Furthermore, the sample of posterior values for

TABLE 9.4

Posterior Estimates of Model Parameters for the Spatial Poisson Regression Model

Effect	Posterior Median Of Associated Parameter	95% Credible Set
Intercept	0.048	(−0.355, 0.408)
% age 65 years or older	3.984	(2.736, 5.330)
Proximity to TCE site	0.152	(0.066, 0.226)
% owner occupied	−0.367	(−0.758, 0.049)

each SMR allows us to calculate the posterior probability that each SMR exceeds a particular threshold (e.g., the posterior probability that a local SMR is larger than 2.0 representing twice the number of cases expected). Figure 9.5 provides a map of the local posterior probabilities of observing a SMR greater than 2.0 for the New York leukemia data. For most of the study area, we see low posterior probability of the local SMR exceeding 2.0, but there are some tracts with fairly high posterior probability, most occurring in the city of Binghamton in the south-central portion and in Syracuse in the north-central portion of the study area. The model-based inference mirrors the scan statistic results in Figure 9.4, but with the additional advantage of explanatory covariates and a more refined identification of particular tracks driving the observed local excesses.

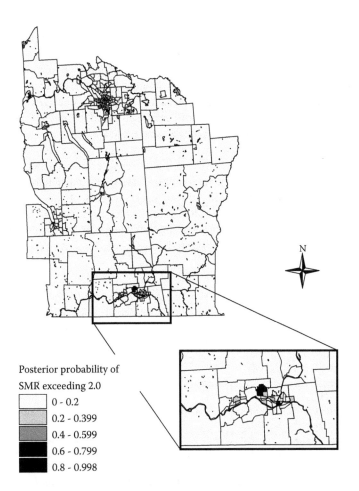

FIGURE 9.5 The posterior probability of the standardized mortality ratio (SMR) exceeding 2.0 in each census tract in the New York leukemia data. Results based on the Poisson regression model with spatially correlated random effects.

9.4 CONCLUSIONS

This chapter provides a brief overview of spatial statistical approaches addressing questions of public health interest within data geocoded to point and area locations. The discussion revealed that the spatial resolution of the data often defines the support provided for different analytical approaches. Also, different statistical approaches often address different research questions of interest, and even the same general set of approaches can perform differently in point and areal data.

To illustrate these points and to review the methods considered, note that both point and areal data support variations of spatial scan statistics to identify the most unusual clusters of events, but the aggregation of events in areal count data results in a loss of spatial resolution, possibly at the expense of missing clusters straddling regional boundaries. Once we move past scan statistics, the sets of analytic methods for point and areal data tend to diverge more dramatically. Analytic methods for point data often focus on statistical estimation of spatial variation in the intensity of events or investigation of nearest-neighbor associations. In contrast, many methods defined for areal count data focus on regression-type models measuring associations between health outcomes and local demographic descriptions from census enumeration districts. In both cases, existing analytic approaches often tend toward slight variations of methods for nonspatial epidemiologic analysis. A need exists for a more central development and classification of spatial statistical methods drawing from a more central set of spatial health hypotheses and models.

The data examples also illustrate how different approaches may yield seemingly contradictory conclusions, yet when viewed with respect to the particular questions addressed and the particular assumptions associated with particular methods, the different methods provide insight into different aspects of the spatial patterns (or lack thereof) in the data. As a result, it is critical for a spatial data analyst to have a toolbox of approaches as well as a working knowledge of the assumptions, capabilities, and limitations of each tool applied.

REFERENCES

1. Maxcy, K. F. An epidemiological study of endemic typhus (Brill's disease) in the southeastern United States with special reference to the mode of transmission. *Public Health Reports* 1926, 41, 2967–2995.
2. Lilienfeld, D. E.; Stolley, P. D. *Foundations of Epidemiology*. 3rd ed. Oxford University Press, New York, 1984.
3. Bailey, T. C.; Gatrell, A. C. *Interactive Spatial Data Analysis*. Addison Wesley Longman, Harlow, Essex, UK, 1995.
4. Diggle, P. J. *Statistical Analysis of Spatial Point Patterns*. 2nd ed. Oxford University Press, New York, 2003.
5. Cressie, N. A. C. *Statistics for Spatial Data*. Rev. ed. Wiley, New York, 1993.
6. Banerjee, S.; Carlin, B. P.; Gelfand, A. E. *Hierarchical Modeling and Analysis for Spatial Data*. Chapman and Hall/CRC Press, Boca Raton, FL, 2004.
7. Schabenberger, O.; Gotway, C. A. *Statistical Methods for Spatial Data Analysis*. Chapman and Hall/CRC Press, Boca Raton, FL, 2005.
8. Besag, J.; Newell, J. The detection of clusters in rare diseases. *Journal of the Royal Statistical Society, Series A* 1991, 154, 327–333.

9. Waller, L. A.; Gotway, C. A. *Applied Spatial Statistics for Public Health Data.* Wiley, Hoboken, NJ, 2004.
10. Diggle, P. J. Overview of statistical methods for disease mapping and its relationship to cluster detection. In *Spatial Epidemiology: Methods and Applications*, Elliott, P.; Wakefield, J. C.; Best, N. G.; Briggs, D. J., Eds. Oxford University Press, Oxford, UK, 1999, pp. 87–103.
11. Cuzick, J.; Edwards, R. Spatial clustering for inhomogeneous populations (with discussion). *Journal of the Royal Statistical Society, Series B* 1990, 52, 73–104.
12. Glaz, J.; Naus, J.; Wallenstein, S. *Scan Statistics.* Springer, New York, 2001.
13. Kulldorff, M. A spatial scan statistic. *Communications in Statistics: Theory and Methods* 1997, 26, 1487–1496.
14. Openshaw, S.; Craft, A. W.; Charlton, M.; Birch, J. M. Investigation of leukaemia clusters by use of a geographical analysis machine. *Lancet* 1988, 1, 272–273.
15. Patil, G. P.; Taillie, C. Upper level set scan statistic for detecting arbitrarily shaped hotspots. *Environmental and Ecological Statistics* 2004, 11, 183–197.
16. Turnbull, B. W.; Iwano, E. J.; Burnett, W. S.; Howe, H. L.; Clark, L. C. Monitoring for clusters of disease: application to leukemia incidence in upstate New York. *American Journal of Epidemiology* 1990, 132 (supplement), S136–S143.
17. Waller, L. A.; Turnbull, B. W.; Clark, L. C.; Nasca, P. Spatial pattern analysis to detect rare disease clusters. In *Case Studies in Biometry*, Lange, N.; Ryan, L.; Billard, L.; Brillinger, D.; Conquest, L.; Greenhouse, J., Eds. Wiley, New York, 1994, pp. 3–23.
18. Anselin, L. *Spatial Econometrics: Methods and Models.* Kluwer Academic, Dordrecht, Netherlands, 1988.
19. New York State Department of Environmental Conservation. *Inactive Hazardous Waste Disposal Sites in New York State.* Vol. 7. New York State Department of Environmental Conservation, Albany, 1987.
20. McCullagh, P.; Nelder, J. A. *Generalized Linear Models.* 2nd ed. Chapman and Hall, New York, 1989.
21. Carlin, B. P.; Louis, T. A. *Bayes and Empirical Bayes Methods for Data Analysis.* 2nd ed. Chapman and Hall/CRC Press, Boca Raton, FL, 2000.
22. Gelman, A.; Carlin, J. B.; Stern, H. S.; Rubin, D. B. *Bayesian Data Analysis.* 2nd ed. Chapman and Hall/CRC Press, Boca Raton, FL, 2004.
23. Clayton, D.; Kaldor, J. Empirical Bayes estimates of age-standardized relative risks for use in disease mapping. *Biometrics* 1987, 43, 671–682.
24. Besag, J.; York, J.; Mollie, A. Bayesian image restoration, with two applications in spatial statistics (with discussion). *Annals of the Institute of Statistical Mathematics* 1991, 43, 1–59.
25. Besag, J. Spatial interaction and the statistical analysis of lattice systems (with discussion). *Journal of the Royal Statistical Society, Series B* 1974, 36, 192–225.
26. Spiegelhalter, D.; Thomas, A.; Best, N.; Lunn, D. *WinBUGS Version 1.4 User's Manual*, Cambridge University, Cambridge, UK, 2003.

10 Statistical Methods for Incompletely and Incorrectly Geocoded Cancer Data

Dale L. Zimmerman

CONTENTS

10.1 INTRODUCTION

The geocodes, or spatial coordinates, of sites where cancer patients live or work may constitute useful information for developing hypotheses about the etiology of the disease and for testing these hypotheses via statistical analyses. Several statistical methods for the analysis of geocoded cancer data were summarized in chapter 9. These included methods for detecting the existence and identifying the locations of spatial clusters of cases and regression methods for relating cancer incidence to spatially varying risk factors. The hallmark of statistical methods such as these is that conclusions drawn from the analysis can be made with quantifiable uncertainty, subject to the assumptions of the underlying probability model on which the analysis is based. An example of such a conclusion is the statement: The probability that we would observe a cancer cluster of this magnitude, if cancer cases occurred totally at random within the at-risk population, is less than .001.

Among the various assumptions of the probability models on which the validity of standard spatial statistical analyses rest, there are two that pertain specifically to geocodes: (1) every case or attribute observation has a geocode assigned to it (complete geocoding), and (2) the geocodes assigned to cases or attribute observations are measured and recorded without error (correct geocoding). These assumptions are rarely, if ever, fully satisfied. In fact, in public health practice it is common for 10%, 20%, or perhaps even 30% of the cases to fail to geocode (incomplete geocoding), and of those cases that do geocode, some may be wrong (incorrect geocoding). For example, Gregorio et al.[1] and Oliver et al.[2] reported on public health studies in which a geocode could not be assigned to 14% and 26%, respectively, of the records in the data set. Krieger et al.[3] conducted an experiment in which four commercial geocoding firms were asked to geocode the same test file of 70 addresses, of which 50 had errors typical of the type seen in practice (e.g., out-of-range address numbers and misspelled street names). They found that the firms' error rates (as measured by the proportion of addresses that were assigned to the wrong census block group geocode) ranged from 16% to 56% on the test file. The firm with the lowest error rate was then given a larger set of addresses randomly selected from public health databases; of these, 5% failed to geocode, and 4% of the remainder were geocoded incorrectly. Furthermore, results given by Cayo and Talbot[4] imply that more than 6% of the rural addresses in an area of upstate New York that geocoded had positional errors greater than 1.0 kilometer. Additional studies of the proportion of incorrect geocodes in health data sets, and of the average distance between the correct and incorrect geocodes, are presented in Dearwent et al.; Bonner et al.; Kravets and Hadden; and Ward et al. [5-8]

In general, incomplete and incorrect geocoding have an adverse effect on a spatial statistical analysis, in particular on the reliability of the conclusions drawn from it. For illustration, consider the map of 100 hypothetical case locations displayed in Figure 10.1. The cases were generated according to a Poisson cluster process (PCP)[9] in the unit square assuming a uniform density for the at-risk population and conditioned on there being 100 cases total. As its name indicates, a PCP generates clusters of cases, with cluster centers following a homogeneous Poisson process. For the particular PCP assumed here, the intensity of clusters is 25 (meaning that the process generates 25 clusters on average in the unit square), the numbers of cases per cluster are independent Poisson random variables with mean 4 (conditioned on their sum being equal to 100), and the locations of cases within a cluster relative to its center are independent random variables with a uniform distribution on a circle of radius 0.1. The visual impression of clustering from Figure 10.1 is strong; hence, we would expect clustering to be detected (with high probability) by any of the plethora of available clustering statistics. Here, we use the Clark-Evans[10] test statistic CE, which is the mean nearest-neighbor distance among cases, normalized to follow approximately a standard normal distribution under the null hypothesis of complete spatial randomness. The value of CE for the data in Figure 10.1 is −3.28, and the two-sided p value associated with this CE is .0010. This constitutes strong evidence of clustering as the p value can be interpreted as the probability, under complete spatial randomness, of obtaining a CE statistic as large or larger (in absolute value) than the one actually obtained for these data.

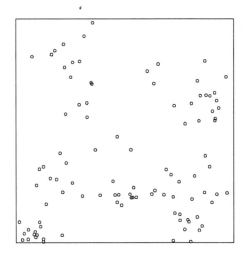

FIGURE 10.1 Hypothetical case locations generated from a Poisson cluster process.

Now consider how the strength of evidence for clustering is affected when either (1) a randomly selected portion of the cases is deleted from the map (mimicking incomplete geocoding), or (2) all cases are perturbed by independent random displacements drawn from the uniform distribution on a circle of radius r centered at 0 (mimicking incorrect geocoding). Three deletion levels (0%, 10%, or 20%) and three perturbation levels ($r = 0$, 0.04, 0.08) were considered. Table 10.1 gives $\overline{CE}$ the average value of CE over 1000 repetitions of the deletion/perturbation scheme, for each of the nine combinations. The p values associated with $\overline{CE}$ are given in parentheses. We observe that $\overline{CE}$ moves toward zero (and thus its associated p value increases) as the geocoding becomes less complete and less accurate, eventually reaching a point at which the evidence for clustering is no longer statistically significant. Indeed, it follows from a well-known result in the theory of point processes[11] that this PCP will converge to a homogeneous Poisson process as r gets arbitrarily large.

Some additional demonstrations and treatments of the effects of incorrect geocoding were provided by Diggle,[12] Jacquez,[13] Waller,[14] Jacquez and Waller,[15] and Burra et al.[16] for point location data and by Gabrosek and Cressie[17] and Cressie and

TABLE 10.1
$\overline{CE}$ for Nine Deletion/Perturbation Combinations

Cases	Perturbation Radius		
	0	0.04	0.08
100	−3.28 (.0010)	−2.83 (.0047)	−1.54 (.1248)
90	−3.13 (.0018)	−2.76 (.0059)	−1.42 (.1571)
80	−2.96 (.0031)	−2.54 (.0111)	−1.34 (.1858)

Kornak[18] for point-level attribute data. Also relevant to the incorrect geocoding problem is the geographic masking methodology of Armstrong, Rushton, and Zimmerman,[19] who studied the effects on statistical analyses of intentionally perturbing the spatial locations to protect the confidentiality of individuals. In contrast, the effects of incomplete geocoding have received virtually no attention.

In this chapter, I review some existing statistical methods for dealing with incompletely and incorrectly geocoded data, and in a few situations for which no methods currently exist I propose some. Unless noted otherwise, I assume that the ZIP codes of all cases, including those that do not geocode, are recorded correctly. This assumption is often nearly satisfied; in chapter 5, for example, Boscoe reported that the ZIP codes for more than 99.99% of incoming cases in the New York Cancer Registry are correctly recorded. One implication of this assumption is that some potentially useful, albeit imprecise, information on location is available for virtually every case.

10.2 ANALYSIS OF INCOMPLETELY GEOCODED DATA

In this section, I focus on methods for analyzing incompletely geocoded data assuming that all the cases that did geocode were correctly geocoded. If there is no concomitant spatial information (e.g., ZIP codes) for the nongeocoded cases, then incompletely geocoded data present a type of problem that statisticians call a *missing data* problem. An extensive body of literature exists on such problems; for a comprehensive treatment, see the work of Little and Rubin.[20] If, on the other hand, ZIP codes are available for the nongeocoded cases, then we are faced with a *coarsened data* problem. A coarse datum refers to an observation that is not the true value of the variable of interest but rather a subset of the sample space in which the true datum lies. In the present context, the missing geocodes are stochastically coarsened in the sense that we are unable to predict perfectly in advance whether any particular case will fail to geocode and thus whether the locational information that will be recorded for any given case will be its latitude and longitude or merely its ZIP code. A considerable body of literature also exists on statistical methods for coarsened data; see, for example, the work of Heitjan and Rubin[21] and Heitjan[22] and the references therein. Unfortunately, none of the missing/coarsened data literature specifically considers spatial data with missing geocodes.

10.2.1 EXCLUSION OF NONGEOCODED CASES

A crucial issue in a missing/coarsened data problem concerns the mechanism that led to some of the observations being missing or coarsened, especially whether an observation is missing/coarsened is related to its value. In the particular situation of incomplete geocoding of point location data, the issue is whether the propensity of an observation to geocode is related to its location or the locations of other observations. If there is no such relationship, then the missing geocodes are said to be missing completely at random, and the same statistical analysis that was contemplated for the complete data will be valid (unbiased) for the *incomplete data*, that is, the data with the nongeocoded cases excluded. In this case, for example, the kernel density estimator of the intensity of a spatial point process computed from the incomplete data would remain asymptotically unbiased, as would the estimated slope coefficient in a logistic regression of cases and controls on the distance to a putative source of increased risk. However, estimates based on the incomplete data will generally be more variable, and tests of hypotheses will be less powerful. The example in section 10.1 illustrated the degradation of power to detect clustering that results from exclusion of more and more cases.

Even more important, if there is a relationship between the locations of observations and their propensities to geocode, then inferences made by applying standard complete data procedures to the incomplete data are susceptible to a type of selection bias, which in this context we call *geographic bias*, following Oliver et al.[2] As an illustration, suppose that the rural addresses in a data set were less likely to geocode than the urban addresses; in fact, a burgeoning body of evidence indicates that this is invariably true, mostly because of the greater use of rural routes and post office boxes in rural areas.[4,7,8,23,24] If the prevalence of a disease were higher among the rural population than among urban dwellers, then the prevalence for the entire population in the region of interest, estimated from only the observations that geocode, would tend to be too small. Note that this bias would persist regardless of how large a sample was taken. An example of geographic bias not necessarily related to rurality was provided by Gilboa et al.[25] They found, in a case-control study of air quality and birth defects in Texas, that incomplete geocoding resulted in a significant underrepresentation of Hispanic women in the study population, and that the association between maternal ethnicity and risk of birth defects was somewhat different for the observations that geocoded than for the observations that failed to geocode.

Complete exclusion from analysis of those cases that do not geocode fails to take advantage of the concomitant ZIP code information that is usually available and thus results in an inefficient and possibly invalid analysis. The remainder of this section describes some alternative approaches that make use of the concomitant information and therefore do not suffer from these shortcomings.

10.2.2 MODELING THE MISSING DATA MECHANISM

If the failure of some cases to geocode is related to their locations, then it may sometimes be possible to meaningfully model or otherwise account for the missing data mechanism (or coarsening mechanism) directly. A guiding principle in this regard could be the evidence, from the literature cited, that nongeocoded cases occur disproportionately in rural areas. Specific implementations of this principle will vary with the type of data (point location, point attribute, or areal attribute) analyzed. In this section, I merely illustrate how this principle might be used to adjust a kernel-smoothing estimator of the intensity of a spatial point process for the occurrence of nongeocoded cases. Further details and generalizations are given in Zimmerman.[26]

Recall the definition of the kernel intensity estimator given in chapter 9:

$$\hat{\lambda}(s) = \sum_{i=1}^{n} K_h(s - s_i) \equiv \sum_{i=1}^{n} h^{-1} K(h^{-1} \| s - s_i \|) \tag{10.1}$$

where $K(\cdot)$ is a univariate symmetric kernel function, and h is the bandwidth. Now, for each point s in the study region D, define a geocoding indicator random variable

$$G(s) = \begin{cases} 1, & \text{if an event at site } s \text{ geocodes} \\ 0, & \text{otherwise.} \end{cases}$$

Also, define a function $\phi(s)$, which we call the *geocoding propensity function*, as follows: $\phi(s) = P\{G(s) = 1\}$. Assume that $\phi(s) > 0$ for all $s \in D$. Note that if $\phi(s)$ is equal to 1.0 across the entire study region, then geocoding is complete, and there is no geographic bias; if $\phi(s)$ varies across the study region, then geocoding tends to be incomplete, and $\hat{\lambda}(s)$ is geographically biased. Observe also that if $\phi(s)$ is less than 1.0 but constant across the study region, then geocoding tends to be incomplete, and $\hat{\lambda}(s)$ is biased, but the bias is not geographic because the intensity estimate is affected equally over the entire study region.

Let $\lambda_I(s)$ denote the intensity function for the process associated with the incompletely geocoded data. In light of Equation 10.1, the natural kernel intensity estimator of $\lambda_I(s)$ is

$$\hat{\lambda}_I(s) = \sum_{\substack{i=1 \\ i \in \mathcal{G}}}^{n} K_h(s - s_i), \tag{10.2}$$

where $\mathcal{G}$ is the set of all cases that geocoded. Although this estimator is asymptotically unbiased for $\lambda_I(s)$, it is biased for the complete data intensity $\lambda(s)$. The relationship between the incomplete-data and complete-data intensity functions can be shown[27] to be

$$\lambda_I(s) = \phi(s)\lambda(s), \tag{10.3}$$

or equivalently that

$$\lambda(s) = \{\phi(s)\}^{-1}\lambda_I(s).$$

This last expression suggests that we might obtain an estimator of $\lambda(s)$ with less geographic bias by inflating each summand in Equation 10.2 as follows:

$$\hat{\lambda}_C(s) = \sum_{\substack{i=1 \\ i \in \mathcal{G}}}^{n} \{\hat{\phi}(s_i)\}^{-1} K_h(s - s_i). \tag{10.4}$$

Here, $\hat{\phi}(s_i)$ is an estimate of the geocoding propensity at s_i, which could be obtained, for example, by specifying a parametric model for $\phi(s)$ and estimating the model's parameters in a manner described next. Note that we have used a subscript C on this estimator to indicate that it makes use of the coarse (ZIP code) data. I demonstrated empirically[26] that the performance of $\hat{\lambda}_C(s)$ is vastly superior to that of $\hat{\lambda}_I(s)$ in the presence of substantial geographic bias.

One simple model for the geocoding propensity function could be based on a dichotomous rural-urban classification of ZIP codes. Suppose that each ZIP code in the geographic region under study can be classified as either urban or rural and suppose we agree to say that a point s is urban or rural according to whether it lies in an urban or rural ZIP code. Suppose further that a case occurring in an urban ZIP code is geocoded with probability ϕ_U; a case occurring in a rural ZIP code is geocoded with probability ϕ_R (where $0 < \phi_U, \phi_R < 1$). We would expect that $\phi_R < \phi_U$, but this is not required. Then, Equation 10.3 can be expressed as

$$\lambda_I(s) = \begin{cases} \phi_U \lambda(s) \text{ if } s \text{ is urban} \\ \phi_R \lambda(s) \text{ if } s \text{ is rural,} \end{cases}$$

and Equation 10.4 can be expressed as

$$\hat{\lambda}_C(s) = \sum_{\substack{i=1 \\ i \in \mathcal{R}}}^{n} \hat{\phi}_R^{-1} K_h(s - s_i) + \sum_{\substack{i=1 \\ i \in \mathcal{U}}}^{n} \hat{\phi}_U^{-1} K_h(s - s_i)$$

where $\{\mathcal{R}, \mathcal{U}\}$ is the partition of $\mathcal{G}$ into subsets of rural and urban ZIP codes, $\hat{\phi}_R$ is the observed proportion of cases in rural ZIP codes that geocode, and $\hat{\phi}_U$ is the observed proportion of cases in urban ZIP codes that geocode.

Specifications of the geocoding propensity based on a dichotomous urban-rural classification can be extended easily for use with a polytomous classification. However, discrete classifications of rurality do not explicitly account for the aforementioned monotonicity (and relative smoothness) of the propensity's relationship with population size or density. As an alternative to assigning geocoding probabilities on the basis of an urban-rural classification, one could consider taking the geocoding propensity to be a continuous, monotone increasing function of the background population density. A natural, parsimonious choice for this function would be the logistic function

$$\phi(s) = \frac{1}{1 + \exp[-\beta_0 - \beta_1 v(s)]}$$

where $v(s)$ represents the background population density at s. For this model, the logit of the geocoding propensity is a linear function of population density, that is,

$$\log\left(\frac{\phi(s)}{1 - \phi(s)}\right) = \beta_0 + \beta_1 v(s), \tag{10.5}$$

but a quadratic function or any other function that is linear in its parameters on the logit scale is permissible. We then have

$$\lambda_I(s) = \frac{\lambda(s)}{1 + \exp[-\beta_0 - \beta_1 v(s)]}.$$

TABLE 10.2

Proportions of NHIS Addresses that Geocoded by Population Size Category

Population Size	Number of Counties	Number of Households	Percentage Geocoded
≥1 million	300	138,281	95.1
250,000–999,999	194	48,992	90.4
50,000–249,999	106	23,379	84.8
20,000–49,999	76	17,625	78.1
2,500–19,999	110	19,805	64.4
< 2,500	48	4,339	43.7

Moreover, if the propensity function is given by Equation 10.5, then Equation 10.4 becomes

$$\hat{\lambda}_C(s) = \sum_{\substack{i=1 \\ i \in \mathcal{G}}}^{n} [1 + \exp\{-\hat{\beta}_0 - \hat{\beta}_1 v(s_i)\}] K_h(s - s_i). \tag{10.6}$$

Here, $v(s_i)$ could be approximated by the population density over the ZIP code (or other areal unit) to which s_i belongs, and β_0 and β_1 may be estimated from a standard logistic regression of the observed geocoding indicator variables on the approximated $v(s_i)$. Note that in the United States, ZIP code densities can be approximated using population and area information available for Zip Code Tabulation Areas (ZCTAs), although the cautionary note of Krieger et al.[28] should be heeded.

To illustrate the plausibility of a logistic specification of geocoding propensity in a real setting, we examine some results obtained by Kravets and Hadden[7] in an analysis of data from the National Health Interview Survey (NHIS), taken from 1995 through 2001. Addresses for a subset of 252,421 households — 89% of all households in the survey — that (1) resided in housing units built before 1990 and (2) were located in 1990 census block groups that could be unambiguously assigned to a 2000 block group using published census block relationship files were submitted to a commercially available geocoding program, and the proportion of addresses to which the program could assign a block group was determined. Kravets and Hadden listed these proportions by the USDA urban-rural continuum code for the enclosing county; the same results are summarized in Table 10.2 in a slightly reduced fashion, using only the population size. More specifically, those codes that have the same population range are pooled, which results in six population size categories: ≥1 million, 250,000–999,999, 50,000–249,999, 20,000–49,999, 2,500–19,999, and <2,500. The proportions of addresses in these categories that geocoded, shown in the rightmost column of Table 10.2, clearly indicate that the geocoding propensity tends to increase with population size.

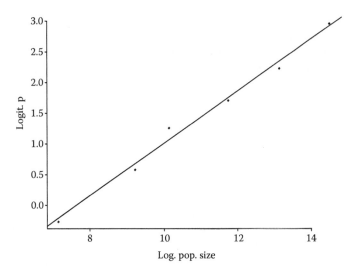

FIGURE 10.2 Plot of logit transform of the geocoding propensity versus the natural logarithm of county population size, for the NHIS data.

In fact, a plot of the log of these proportions versus the log population size (Figure 10.2) appears quite linear, which suggests fitting a logistic regression model of propensity on log population size, that is, $\log[\phi(s)/\{1-\phi(s)\}] = \gamma_0 + \gamma_1 \log\{v(s)\}$. Such a model was fitted by standard logistic regression methods (using half the upper limit of each population category as a proxy for the population size except for the largest category, for which 2 million was the proxy) and is drawn in Figure 10.2.

Although a model that is linear in its parameters on the logit scale provides a good fit to the observed NHIS geocoded proportions, this may not always be so. Therefore, it is worth noting that an even more general way to model the dependence of the geocoding propensity on population density is to assume only that $\phi(s) = (1 + \exp[-\gamma_0 - f\{v(s)\}])^{-1}$, where $f(\cdot)$ is an unspecified smooth function. The $\phi(s_i)$ may be estimated using the fitted nonparametric logistic regression of the g_i on the $v(s_i)$.

10.2.3 PSEUDOCODING

A third approach for dealing with incomplete geocoding is to assign approximate geocodes, or *pseudocodes*, to the nongeocoded cases. These assignments can be made either deterministically or stochastically. In the terminology of statistical methodology for missing data problems, such assignments are called *imputations*.

Perhaps the simplest deterministic pseudocoding method is to assign each nongeocoded case to the centroid of the ZIP code in which it resides or to the centroid of all geocoded cases in that ZIP code; however, there are at least two serious problems associated with this. First, the centroid may not be representative of where the population in that ZIP code actually lives; indeed, the centroid may lie in a completely uninhabited portion of the ZIP code. Although this problem may be mitigated by replacing the ordinary centroid with a population-weighted centroid, it is not eliminated altogether. Second, multiple nongeocoded cases in the same ZIP code will be assigned exactly the same pseudocode, possibly resulting in a spurious cluster. Thus, this method may not be appropriate in conjunction with certain clustering or cluster identification investigations. On the other hand, trend surface analysis and other spatial regression analyses may still go forward, provided that the modeler includes a nugget effect in the residual covariance structure of the regression model. The inclusion of a nugget effect allows for variability among distinct replicate attributes at the centroid. A spatial regression analysis of data that includes deterministically pseudocoded cases should nonetheless account for the uncertainty of the actual locations of pseudocoded cases (see section 10.3).

As for stochastic methods of pseudocoding, there are several possibilities. One could, for example, assign nongeocoded cases according to some continuous probability distribution with support that is limited to the ZIP code's geographic extent. Possible distributions would include the uniform distribution, a truncated bivariate normal distribution with mean at the ZIP code centroid, or a smooth, normalized approximation to the population density over the ZIP code. Alternatively, one could make these assignments according to a discrete uniform distribution with support on the point locations of cases in the ZIP code that did geocode, which is a form of a general technique known as *hot deck imputation*. Although this second method naturally accounts for population density and may be somewhat simpler to implement than the first, it is also more likely to create a spurious cluster. Both methods could be modified to take information on demographic covariates into account. Moreover, multiple assignments could be made for each case, analogous to the notion of multiple imputation in missing data methodology.

The foregoing makes it clear that pseudocoding, whether deterministic or stochastic, results in a set of data having some geocoding (positional) errors. Thus, to perform an appropriate statistical analysis of such data, we are led to consider statistical methods for handling data with geocoding errors, even if all of the genuinely geocoded cases were geocoded without error. The only difference is that, with pseudocoded data, we know *a priori* which cases are incorrectly geocoded; with completely but incorrectly geocoded data, we generally do not. I therefore combine, in the next section, the presentation of statistical methods for analyzing pseudocoded data with the presentation of methods for analyzing incorrectly geocoded data.

10.3 ANALYSIS OF INCORRECTLY GEOCODED DATA

In this section, the data are assumed to be completely geocoded (possibly as a result of pseudocoding the cases that did not originally geocode), and I focus on the problem of incorrect geocoding. The effect that geocoding errors of sufficient magnitude can have on spatial statistical inference was illustrated in section 10.1. Unfortunately, little research has been published on statistical methods for adjusting inferences to account for these errors. For the analysis of areal-level attribute data, the effects of geocoding errors are minimal if the areal units of analysis are at the ZIP code level or larger. Therefore, what little work has been done on incorrect geocoding has focused on point location and point-level attribute data.

10.3.1 POINT LOCATION DATA

In the case of point location data, Diggle[12] considered how to modify the K function when there are geocoding errors. The K function $K(h)$ of a stationary spatial point process is defined as the expected number of additional events within distance h of an arbitrarily chosen event divided by the expected number of events per unit area, and it is a useful tool for detecting clustering in populations otherwise consistent with complete spatial randomness. However, in cancer studies the at-risk population intensity is nearly always spatially varying, which renders inference based on the ordinary K function ineffectual. A nonstationary analogue of the K function was developed by Baddeley, Möller, and Waagepetersen,[29] but modifications to it that account for geocoding errors have yet to be developed. Therefore, we turn our attention away from the K function to a testing procedure for clustering that does account for inhomogeneity of the at-risk population, the Cuzick-Edwards[30] case-control test.

In the Cuzick-Edwards testing procedure, first the cases are geocoded or pseudocoded and then a number of controls are randomly selected from the at-risk population over the same geographic region; likewise, these are geocoded or pseudocoded. Next, the number of cases that have other cases (rather than controls) as their nearest neighbors is determined, yielding a count T_1; more generally, we determine T_k, the number of cases among the K nearest neighbors of all cases, for selected values of k. A "large" value of T_k indicates that there are more clusters consisting of $K + 1$ cases than can be explained merely by any "background clustering" of the at-risk population. To judge statistical significance, we can compare a normalized statistic, $[T_k - E(T_k)] / \sqrt{\operatorname{var}(T_k)}$, to a chosen percentile from a standard normal distribution; expressions for $E(T_k)$ and $\operatorname{var}(T_k)$ can be found in the work of Cuzick and Edwards.[30] This approach works well if the data are perfectly geocoded, but if some of the cases or controls are pseudocoded by assigning them to, say, ZIP code centroids, then it may be impossible to determine whether the nearest neighbor of a given case is another case or a control, and thus the procedure breaks down (see Figure 10.3). For such a situation, Jacquez[31] developed a method for placing bounds about the true but unobserved value of T_k and about the corresponding true but unobserved p value. Jacquez's method is based on enumerating all the ways in which the coincident pseudocodes may be resolved. Actually, only two resolutions need to be considered: one that always treats a case as the nearest neighbor and another that always treats a control as the nearest neighbor. For evaluating significance, Jacquez suggested that we reject the null hypothesis of no clustering when the upper and lower bounds on the p value are both significant, accept the null hypothesis when neither bound is significant, and withhold judgment when the upper bound is significant but the lower bound is not.

As a final illustration of accounting for geocoding errors in the analysis of point location data, consider the classical spatial epidemiological problem of estimating the intensity of a Poisson spatial point process by the method of maximum likelihood.

FIGURE 10.3 Depiction of coincident pseudo-codes and their effect on the Cuzick-Edwards statistic. Actual but unobserved geocodes of cases and controls are represented by an open circle and a closed circle, respectively, and the pseudo-code (the areal centroid) is represented by an ×. Here, the cases have each other as their nearest neighbors, so the true but unobserved contribution to T_1 from this area would be 2.

Thus, assume that the underlying point process is Poisson, with an intensity function that belongs to a parametric family $\{\lambda_\theta(x,y) : \theta \in \Theta\}$. For this family, the likelihood function associated with a sample $\{(x_i, y_i) : i = 1,...,n\}$ of observed locations in a study area D is, in the absence of geocoding errors, proportional to[9]

$$L(\theta; \{(x_i, y_i) : i = 1,...,n\}) = \exp\left\{-\int_D \lambda_\theta(s,t)\, ds\, dt\right\}\left\{\prod_{i=1}^{n} \lambda_\theta(x_i, y_i)\right\}.$$

A maximum likelihood estimate of θ is a value $\hat{\theta}$ that maximizes L. Now suppose that we do not actually observe the true locations $\{(x_i, y_i) : i = 1,...,n\}$, but instead we observe perturbed versions of them, denoted as $\{(u_i, v_i) : i = 1,...,n\}$. Suppose further that conditional on the true locations, each perturbed location is an independent realization from a distribution with probability density function $f_i((u_i, v_i) \mid (x_i, y_i))$, which is centered at the corresponding true location. In general, there are no restrictions on the form of this probability density function. Zimmerman et al.[32] found that bivariate t densities and mixtures thereof were good candidates for the density of positional errors of rural addresses in an Iowa county, but further research is needed to determine which forms are plausible in other settings. For simplicity of illustration here, we take the geocoding error distributions to be bivariate normal, with means (x_i, y_i), common variances σ^2 (for both components), and correlation zero. Then, if we ignore any available ZIP code information, the joint likelihood of the true and perturbed locations is proportional to the product of $L(\theta; \{(x_i, y_i) : i = 1, \ldots, n\}$ and these bivariate normal densities; furthermore, the unconditional joint likelihood of the perturbed locations is obtained by integrating over the distribution of the true locations and hence is proportional to

$$L^*(\theta, \sigma^2; \{(u_i, v_i) : i = 1, \ldots, n\}$$

$$= (\sigma^2)^{-n} \exp\left\{-\int_D \lambda_\theta(s, t) ds\ dt\right\} \int \int \ldots \int \left\{\prod_{i=1}^n \lambda_\theta(x_i, y_i)\right\}$$

$$\times \exp\left\{-\frac{1}{2\sigma^2} \sum_{i=1}^n [(u_i - x_i)^2 + (v_i - y_i)^2]\right\} dx_1 dy_1 \cdots dx_n dy_n.$$

A geocoding-error-adjusted maximum likelihood estimate of θ is the first part of any value $(\hat{\theta}^*, \hat{\sigma}^2)$ that maximizes L^*. In most practical situations, the integral in L^* cannot be evaluated explicitly, and the likelihood equations do not yield an explicit solution. Therefore, numerical techniques (e.g., numerical integration and Newton–Raphson algorithms) would generally be needed to obtain a maximum likelihood estimate. Further details, modifications for nonnormal geocoding error distributions, and extensions to relative risk estimation from case-control data can be found in Zimmerman and Sun.[33]

10.3.2 POINT-LEVEL ATTRIBUTE DATA

In the case of point-level attribute data, there is a close connection between models for incorrectly geocoded data and the broad family of models that statisticians call *measurement error models*. Cressie and Kornak[18] exploited this connection and described two fundamentally different location error models. In the *coordinate-positioning model*, the investigator's intention is to take attribute observations at preselected sites (e.g., perhaps sites on a regular grid), but because of imprecise positioning instruments, positional coordinate rounding, human error, and so on, the sites where observations are actually taken are perturbed and thus unknown. In the *feature-positioning model*, the investigator records the locations of well-defined features or outcomes (e.g., residences of newly diagnosed cancer patients), but again these locations are not ascertained perfectly. The distinction between the two models pertains to what is known about the means of the location distributions corresponding to the observations. In the first model, these mean locations are known, but in the second model they are unknown. For location errors generated by the coordinate-positioning model, Cressie and Kornak[18] developed appropriate methods for adjusting estimates of spatial trend and spatial covariances and for modifying predictions of attribute values at unsampled locations. No analogous methods of adjustment have been developed for the feature-positioning model, which is unfortunate because it is the more relevant of the two models for geocoded cancer data. It would be particularly useful, for instance, to be able to adjust inference on the coefficients of spatial regression models for relating imprecisely located cancer cases to spatially varying risk factors.

10.4 CONCLUSIONS

This chapter summarized the existing literature, scant as it may be, on methods for analyzing incompletely and incorrectly geocoded cancer data. For a few important problems for which it appears that no methods currently exist, I have made some proposals. More thorough consideration of these and other proposals awaits further research.

In public health surveillance, the geocode is typically regarded as the place where a health event and its causative exposure occur, and it is common practice to use the corresponding individual's place of residence as the geocode. Of course, this is a gross oversimplification. People may be exposed to disease vectors or carcinogens, for example, in their workplaces, in transit, or at other locations. Furthermore, for diseases such as cancer, for which onset may occur years after exposure, the person's place of residence and occupation in the past may be of equal or greater relevance than their geocode at diagnosis. Therefore, it must be noted that no matter how sophisticated and powerful a method of statistical analysis may be at adjusting for the effects of incomplete and incorrect geocoding, it will not reflect the inherent uncertainty associated with using the geocode to represent the location of exposure. However, methods for adjusting inferences for the effects of incorrect geocoding may also be adapted for dealing with data for which regions, rather than points, are used to represent the locations of exposure (see the work of Jacquez et al.[34]).

ACKNOWLEDGMENT

This chapter is based on research made possible through a cooperative agreement between the Centers for Disease Control and Prevention (CDC) and the Association of Schools of Public Health (ASPH), award number S-3111; its contents are the responsibility of the author and do not necessarily reflect the official views of the CDC or ASPH.

REFERENCES

1. Gregorio, D. I., et al. Subject loss in spatial analysis of breast cancer. *Health and Place*, 5, 173–177, 1999.
2. Oliver, M. N., et al. Geographic bias related to geocoding in epidemiologic studies. *International Journal of Health Geographics*, 4, 29, 2005.
3. Krieger, N., et al. On the wrong side of the tracts? Evaluating the accuracy of geocoding in public health research. *American Journal of Public Health*, 91, 1114–1116, 2001.
4. Cayo, M. R., and Talbot, T. O. Positional error in automated geocoding of residential addresses. *International Journal of Health Geographics*, 2, 10, 2003.
5. Dearwent, S. M., Jacobs, R. R., and Halbert, J. B. Locational uncertainty in georeferencing public health datasets. *Journal of Exposure Analysis and Environmental Epidemiology*, 11, 329–334, 2001.
6. Bonner, M. R., et al. Positional accuracy of geocoded addresses in epidemiologic research. *Epidemiology*, 14, 408–412, 2003.
7. Kravets, N., and Hadden, W. C. The accuracy of address coding and the effects of coding errors. *Health and Place*, 13, 293–298, 2007.

8. Ward, M. H., et al. Positional accuracy of two methods of geocoding. *Epidemiology*, 16, 542–547, 2005.

9. Diggle, P. J. *Statistical Analysis of Spatial Point Patterns*. Arnold, London, 2003, p. 64.

10. Clark, P. J., and Evans, F. C. Distance to nearest neighbor as a measure of spatial relationships in populations. *Ecology*, 35, 23–30, 1954.

11. Cox, D. R., and Isham, V. *Point Processes*, Chapman and Hall, London, 1980.

12. Diggle, P. J. Point process modelling in epidemiology. In *Statistics for the Environment,* Barnett, V., and Turkman, K. F., Eds., Wiley, New York, 1993, p. 89–110.

13. Jacquez, G. M. Disease cluster statistics for imprecise space-time locations. *Statistics in Medicine*, 15, 873–885, 1996.

14. Waller, L. A. Statistical power and design of focused clustering studies. *Statistics in Medicine*, 15, 765–782, 1996.

15. Jacquez, G. M., and Waller, L. A. The effect of uncertain locations on disease cluster statistics. In *Quantifying Spatial Uncertainty in Natural Resources: Theory and Applications for GIS and Remote Sensing*, Mowrer, H. T., and Congalton, R. G., Eds., Ann Arbor Press, Chelsea, MI, 2000, p. 53–64.

16. Burra, T., et al., Conceptual and practical issues in the detection of local disease clusters: a study of mortality in Hamilton, Ontario. *The Canadian Geographer*, 46, 160–171, 2002.

17. Gabrosek, J., and Cressie, N. The effect on attribute prediction of location uncertainty in spatial data. *Geographical Analysis*, 34, 262–285, 2002.

18. Cressie, N., and Kornak, J., Spatial statistics in the presence of location error with an application to remote sensing of the environment. *Statistical Science*, 18, 436–456, 2003.

19. Armstrong, M. P., Rushton, G., and Zimmerman, D. L. Geographically masking health data to preserve confidentiality. *Statistics in Medicine*, 18, 497–525, 1999.

20. Little, R. J. A., and Rubin, D. B. *Statistical Analysis with Missing Data*, 2nd ed., Wiley, Hoboken, NJ, 2002.

21. Heitjan, D. F., and Rubin, D. B. Ignorability and coarse data. *Annals of Statistics*, 19, 2244–2253, 1991.

22. Heitjan, D. F. Ignorability and coarse data: some biomedical examples. *Biometrics*, 49, 1099–1109, 1993.

23. Vine, M. F., Degnan, D., and Hanchette, C. Geographic information systems: their use in environmental epidemiologic research. *Environmental Health Perspectives*, 105, 598–605, 1997.

24. McElroy, J. A., et al., Geocoding addresses from a large population-based study: lessons learned. *Epidemiology*, 14, 399–407, 2003.

25. Gilboa, S. M., et al., Comparison of residential geocoding methods in population-based study of air quality and birth defects. *Environmental Research*, 101, 256–262, 2006.

26. Zimmerman, D. L. Estimating the intensity of a spatial point process from locations coarsened by incomplete geocoding. *Biometrics* (in press).

27. Stoyan, D., Kendall, W. S., and Mecke, J. *Stochastic Geometry and Its Applications*. Wiley, Chichester, 1987.

28. Krieger, N., et al. ZIP code caveat: bias due to spatiotemporal mismatches between ZIP codes and U.S. Census-defined geographic areas—the public health disparities geocoding project. *American Journal of Public Health*, 92, 1100–1102, 2002.

29. Baddeley, A. J., Möller, J., and Waagepetersen, R. Non- and semi-parametric estimation of interaction in inhomogeneous point patterns. *Statistica Neerlandica*, 54, 329–358, 2000.

30. Cuzick, J., and Edwards, R. Spatial clustering for inhomogeneous populations. *Journal of the Royal Statistical Society, Series B*, 52, 73–104, 1990.

31. Jacquez, G. M. Cuzick and Edwards' test when exact locations are unknown. *American Journal of Epidemiology*, 140, 58–64, 1994.

32. Zimmerman, D. L., et al., Modeling the probability distribution of positional errors incurred by residential address geocoding. *International Journal of Health Geographics*, 6, 1, 2007.

33. Zimmerman, D. L., and Sun, P. *Estimating Spatial Intensity and Variation in Relative Risk from Locations Subject to Geocoding Errors* (Technical Report 363). Department of Statistics, University of Iowa, 2006.

34. Jacquez, G. M., et al. Global, local, and focused geographic clustering for case-control data with residential histories. *Environmental Health: A Global Access Science Source*, 4, 4, 2005.

11 Using Geocodes to Estimate Distances and Geographic Accessibility for Cancer Prevention and Control

Marc Armstrong, Barry R. Greene, and Gerard Rushton

CONTENTS

11.1 INTRODUCTION

The accuracy of estimated distances from people to facilities depends on the quality of the geocodes describing people, facilities, and the geospatial data used to link the two. For example, a simple case occurs when people are defined by the latitude and longitude coordinate of their residence; facilities are also defined in the same coordinate system, and the geospatial data used to link the two are covered by equations describing the spherical earth.[1] Other distance metrics, as described in section 11.2, are also often used.

11.2 DISTANCE METRICS AND CALCULATION METHODS

Distances play important roles in many types of geographical analyses of health information. For example, distance is an essential component in linking both individuals and groups to sources of exposure to environmental contaminants; distance also plays a key role in accessibility to and choice of health services. Such distances may be calculated between individual points (e.g., residence location and screening facility), as well as between areas (e.g., between census tracts) and between points and areas (demand measured as a population in a tract and a health care facility). Moreover, distances can be computed using simple interpoint distances or more complex distance computations that are made using summations of link distances computed using a digital representation of a transportation network.

11.2.1 INTERPOINT DISTANCES

When it is assumed that travel is not restricted to a network or that a network has straight-line connections among places, then the Euclidean (or "crow fly") metric can be used. This metric, however, is simply a special case of the more generic Minkowski metric, which is specified as

$$d(a, b) = (|a_1 - b_1|^p + |a_2 - b_2|^p)^{1/p},$$

where $p \geq 1$, $d(a, b)$ is the distance from a to b, and $a = (a_1, a_2)$ and $b = (b_1, b_2)$ are points in a Cartesian coordinate system.

Given two points a and b, the Euclidean metric distance between them is specified as

$$d_e(a, b) = (|a_1 - b_1|^2 + |a_2 - b_2|^2)^{1/2}.$$

There are many examples of distances computed using this method.[2–4] In some applications and in some areas, travel is restricted to rectilinear transportation links. For example, movement through many metropolitan areas is restricted to straight blocks that meet at orthogonal intersections. In such cases, the Manhattan metric may be more appropriate to use.

$$d_m(a, b) = (|a_1 - b_1| + |a_2 - b_2|), \quad \text{that is,} \quad p = 1.$$

When data are represented using spherical coordinates, such as latitude and longitude, and when distances must be computed over large portions of the earth, it is appropriate to use distance calculations that are based on spherical trigonometry.

$$d_s(a, b) = \cos^{-1} (\cos a \cos b + \sin a \sin b \cos A)$$

where a and b represent colatitude (90– latitude) values for two points that are separated by longitude difference A. The Euclidean, Manhattan, and spherical metrics are useful for situations in which spatial interaction is predictably well defined by straight-line connections. In most instances, however, real interaction occurs in less-regular ways, as in cases where transportation networks are the basis of interaction. Several approaches are available to introduce increased realism into the distance estimation process. The first involves the use of a parameter to inflate distances to (usually) greater than Euclidean, but less than Manhattan.

$$d_k(a, b) = k\,(|a_1 - b_1|^2 + |a_2 - b_2|^2)^{1/2}, \quad k \geq 1$$

In this case, Euclidean distance is multiplied by a parameter k to inflate the estimated value. In other cases, the value of p in the Minkowski metric as described is also modified.

$$d_{k,p}(a, b) = k(|a_1 - b_1|^p + |a_2 - b_2|^p)^{1/p}$$

where k and p are empirically derived parameters typically estimated using models that, for a sample of locations, use "known" interpoint distances derived from high-accuracy sources. Once k and p are estimated, they are applied for all other point-to-point distance calculations in an area. The use of these parametric distances, however, assumes that the road density and configuration remain constant throughout an area of interest. For an extended discussion of distance estimation methods, see chapter 10 in the work of Love et al.[5] Phibbs and Luft investigated relationships between straight-line distances and travel times for a sample of patient visits to health facilities.[6]

11.2.2 Network Distances

The parametric distances described are used to approximate distances that would be obtained if a network were available. With the widespread availability of networks in the form of digital line graphs, TIGER (Topologically Integrated Geographic Encoding and Referencing) line files, and other sources, the computation of network distances has become more common.[7,8] Such distances are computed by specifying starting and ending points (e.g., residence and health care facility) and summing distances along intermediate links between them. The intermediate links are specified typically using assumptions about travel behavior through the network. The shortest path is often used, although other transformations, such as shortest time, are used if necessary link attributes are present.

11.2.2.1 Networks

A network can be conceptualized as a directed graph. A directed graph is indicated, in this case, because travel restrictions are commonly employed in transportation networks (e.g., one-way streets). Each link in the graph can be represented as a straight-line segment or, more commonly, as a chain of points that approximates its real geometry.

The length of the chain is determined by summing its interpoint distances.

$$L = \sum_{i=1}^{npts} ((a_{1i} - b_{1i})^2 + (a_{2i} - b_{2i})^2)^{1/2}$$

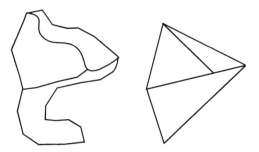

FIGURE 11.1 A network with curvature that is abstracted into a line graph.

11.2.2.2 Link Attributes

Links may have one or more attributes associated with them. Although length for straight-line segments can be calculated, if multiple traversals of a network will be performed, then it is often more cost-effective to compute lengths and store them as an attribute. In a similar way, links can have other attributes, such as speed limits, traversal times (including multiple times based on time of day), or other measures of effort. Such measures might be based, for example, on slope, energy requirements, or some other impedance factor. These attributes can be substituted for distance in shortest-path algorithms to minimize transit time or total energy expenditures.

Digital representations of road networks are widely available and form an integral part of the U.S. national spatial data infrastructure. Such networks can play an important role in the analysis of health information and are particularly important in the calculation of distance relations. A network can be abstracted from its real complexity to an abstract representation using a graph (Figure 11.1).

For a graph to be useful in analyses, it must be structured. One way to impose needed structure is to label elements of a graph and record topological (adjacency and connectivity) information. Figure 11.2 shows a labeled network that consists of 10 nodes linked by 15 edges.

A graph can be represented using a table that records nodes and edges (links). This graph is then represented as a table that shows the direct links between nodes along with the distance associated with the edge. Note that there are zeros along the diagonal, and the matrix is symmetrical about the diagonal, indicating that the impedances are transitive. If there were other factors, such as elevation or another indicator of effort, then the matrix would be asymmetrical.

As can be seen in Figure 11.3, most adjacency matrices are sparse and are inefficient storage and analysis structures. As a consequence, alternative representations have been developed. Figure 11.4 shows a reduced version of Figure 11.3 in which each row represents a node and lists those nodes that connect to it as well as the distance along the link formed by the two nodes.

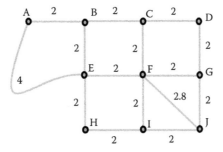

FIGURE 11.2 A simple network with nodes and links. Nodes are identified by letters. Link impedances are indicated by numbers.

	A	B	C	D	E	F	G	H	I	J
A	0	2			4					
B	2	0	2		2					
C		2	0	2		2				
D			2	0			2			
E	4	2			0	2		2		
F			2		2	0	2		2	2.8
G				2		2	0			2
H					2			0	2	
I						2		2	0	2
J						2.8	2		2	0

FIGURE 11.3 An adjacency matrix for the graph shown in Figure 11.2.

A	B 2	E 4			
B	A 2	C 2	E 2		
C	B 2	D 2	F 2		
D	C 2	G 2			
E	A 4	B 2	F 2	H 2	
F	C 2	E 2	G 2	I 2	J 2.8
G	D 2	F 2	J 2		
H	E 2	I 2			
I	F 2	H 2	J 2		
J	F 2.8	G 2	I 2		

FIGURE 11.4 A reduced form of the adjacency matrix shown in Figure 3.

11.3 SPATIAL AGGREGATION EFFECTS: ESTIMATING DISTANCES WHEN PEOPLE ARE REPRESENTED BY AREAS

Often, geographic coordinates are not available for individuals and facilities; instead, geocodes are available for areas. For example, distance estimates are required between points (e.g., the locations of health care providers) and areas (e.g., demands for service aggregated to census units). The distance from a point to a polygon can be specified as a distance from that point to the closest polygon vertex or face. To determine the closest part of the line or polygon to a point, the distance must be calculated between it and each point of a line segment that defines the line or polygon boundary. Alternatively, distances can be calculated between the point and the centroid of the polygon. This centroid can be either the geometric center or a weighted center that takes into consideration the internal distribution of some attribute. The choice is usually dependent on the assumptions made for a particular application.

Centroids are often computed and stored as components of the data structures used by geographic information system (GIS) software. Such locations are used, for example, to define the location of labels for polygons. These points can therefore be accessed and used in analyses. When GIS software is not used, the geometric centroid can be specified for regular polygons as the mean of the x and y coordinate values. For polygons that have irregular concave and convex shapes, an alternative approach to calculation is required.

It is common to know the locations of facilities, although, perhaps surprisingly, there are few standards for uniquely identifying the location of health facilities around the world.[9] Distances are estimated by applying the methods discussed in section 11.2 to the centroids of the defined areas (e.g., ZIP codes, postal codes, census tracts, counties) using methods discussed in section 11.2. Although these distances are estimates, there are several interesting properties we know about them. If we are interested in the maximum distance people are from their closest facility, then estimates made in this way usually will be underestimates of the true maximum distances because using a centroid will result in distances for some people in the area to be underestimated and the distances of others to be overestimated. In general, it is known that if geometric centroids are used, then distances are generally underestimated by this method when distances are estimated to just one facility.[10–12] However, when more than one facility is involved, it is not known whether distances are over- or underestimated, except that the error increases as the ratio of the number of aggregated areas divided by the number of facilities decreases.[13,14] As the average size of the aggregated areas increases, relative to the number of facilities, the distance estimation errors increase. It follows that representing people by the smallest areas for which data exists is preferred. Francis et al. provided advice on this question, where q is the number of areas representing the population distribution and p represents the number of facilities serving the people:

> Anyone using procedures to estimate distances from dispersed demand to facilities based on spatial aggregations of the demand can use the parameter q/p to estimate whether unacceptable levels of error might exist in the results of their analyses. Such analysis systems could alert users when they make distance estimates within the domain of the parameter q/p where measurement errors are now known to increase rapidly.[13] (p. 84)

When there is concern about the error that results from estimating distances from people located in areas to facilities, it is possible to reduce this error by disaggregating the population to smaller areas and representing the spatial pattern of people by the smaller areas.[15,16]

11.4 MEASURING GEOGRAPHIC ACCESSIBILITY

Geographic accessibility is measured in a variety of ways.[2,17] The most straightforward measure is the distance of a person to that person's closest health facility.[4] A common GIS function partitions space into areas that are closest to a given set of facilities. Adding a hypothetical new facility can quickly show how areas that are far from a health facility would be affected. Location-allocation methods, recently incorporated in several commercial GIS software releases, find optimal locations for facilities that can be used to select locations that are optimal with respect to defined objectives. Typical objectives are to minimize total travel distance from people to their closest facility, to minimize the maximum distance of people to their closest facility, or to optimize multiple criteria.[18] These methods are often incorporated in spatial decision support systems to assist people who are making location decisions for health facilities.[19–21] They have also been extended and adapted to address the problem of optimal routing of services[22] and of simulating alternative locations for health services.[23] Use of optimal location methods for locating health facilities has been extensively discussed.[24–27] Liu and Zhu in 2004 developed software ACCESS integrated with GIS to support the process of accessibility analysis within urban settings.[28] Algorithms for measuring accessibility to potential users of facilities have been developed for competing health

facilities; people make spatial choices of the facilities based on the relative characteristics of the facilities as well as their relative distances.[29,30] These methods are based
on models of spatial interaction in regional science.[31,32]

Especially for poor populations, geographic accessibility is best measured as the ability to reach health services by public transportation. To answer such questions, it is necessary to code public transportation routes and times and then to geocode the population
in relation to their access to points of service on the public transit routes. Examples can
be found in the work of Lovett et al. and Weber and Kwan.[33,34] It has become common to
identify spatial opportunities within the context of an abstract space-time prism within
which people typically live and work.[35–40] Other studies assessed the impact of travel on
cancer patients' experiences of treatment.[41]

Distances are measured to determine their effects on the spatial choices of people in selecting the place of service that frequently is not the closest place that offers
the service.[29] In urban areas in the United States, measures of accessibility to service
facilities have been shown to be related to spatial structures.[42]

Studies have examined inequities in accessibility of different social groups to
health facilities.[43] Other studies have measured the accessibility potential to the critical mix of health services for colorectal cancer diagnosis and treatment. *Accessibility potential* in the geography literature refers to the inverse distance weighted
access measure that a person experiences in accessing the mix of services they are
likely to need in diagnosis and treatment for a health service. Each element of the
service is measured and often weighted by its importance in the mix. The access
of a person is then measured as directly related to its score in the element mix and
inversely related to the person's distance to the closest occurrence of it. Different
elements of the mix of services are then summed for the person in question to give
a total accessibility score.

11.5 MAPPING GEOGRAPHICAL ACCESSIBILITY

The allocation of demand for services to the location of service providers can be
illustrated using a variety of methods.[44] For example, spider maps show straight-
line connections between supply and demand locations. Network spider maps also
show this relationship but link supply and demand locations using shortest paths
through a network. Geographic accessibility issues are often most clearly seen by
mapping people, disease rates, and facilities.[45,46] Simply locating facilities on a map
and showing areas covered by the facilities within given distances can be an effective way to draw attention to areas that have unusually low levels of access to facilities. Examples can be seen in the literature.[2,20,33,35,47,48] Often, cumulative frequency
graphs and related tables show proportions of people within given distances of their
closest facilities.[2,49] Travel times to facilities are often shown by isochrones — lines
joining points of equal travel distance from a given facility or place.[50]

A common reason for mapping geographical accessibility measures is to identify
areas of health resource shortages. The conventional method was to map ratios of
people per unit of resource. Number of persons per physician is a classic example[51];
more recently, radiation therapy facilities per 1000 cancer cases have been used.[47]
These measures, however, are now out of favor because of the criticism that they

ignore the capability of people outside the measurement area for receiving services from providers within it, as well as people inside the area for receiving services outside. A method that deals with this criticism to some degree is the *floating catchment method*, which measures population per resource unit for a spatial area that is consecutively centered on points on a spatial grid. The result is a spatial surface of accessibility of people to resources. Different maps can show the surface for areas of different size, thus showing how accessibility to resources changes at different spatial scales. Examples can be found in the literature.[35,52-55] To be effective, however, this approach requires that population and resource data are geocoded for small spatial units; also, several common GIS functions are needed to implement the method. ZIP codes, census block groups, or individual facility and people geocodes were used in the research cited. Geovisualization techniques for showing potential opportunities for access to health services in an urban environment have been developed.[56]

11.6 ACCESSIBILITY, DISTANCE, AND EFFECT ON CANCER SCREENING AND TREATMENT

An important reason to estimate distances is to use them to answer questions that arise in cancer research or in cancer prevention and control. Most of these questions relate to the accessibility of people to resources for prevention or treatment.[57] For a long time, it has been known that health-seeking behavior is sensitive to the accessibility of people to health facilities.[58,59] Where facilities are located conveniently to people, they are likely to be used more frequently and especially likely to be used for preventive activities.[60-62] Investigators in Florida found that the degree to which a woman had to travel to a radiation facility lowered the odds of her receiving breast-conserving surgery with radiation.[63] By receiving pretreatment counseling and facilitating access to radiation therapy facilities, the odds of a woman receiving breast-conserving radiation and surgery were increased. In a study of all women residents of New Hampshire who were diagnosed with stage I or II breast cancer, the researchers found that women with early-stage breast cancer were less likely to choose breast-conserving surgery if these women lived 20 or more miles from a radiation treatment facility, and if the diagnosis was made during the winter season the women would forgo radiation treatment because of the difficulty of traveling for radiation in the winter.[64] A similar result was found by Nattinger et al.[65] Among Hispanic, black, and older women and the uninsured, the odds of receiving breast-conserving surgery with radiation fell significantly for every 5-mile increase in distance to a radiation treatment center.[63] Similarly, Rushton and West[66] showed that women diagnosed with localized breast cancer in Iowa were more likely to select mastectomy treatment the further they were from a radiation facility — a conclusion confirmed by Athas et al., who computed the log odds of receiving radiation therapy following breast-conserving surgery for early-stage breast cancer as a function of the square root of travel distance. Distances were computed as network distances from geocoded locations of patients and facilities in a GIS.[66,67]

Punglia and colleagues studied the effect of distance to the nearest radiation treatment facility on the use of postmastectomy radiation therapy (PMRT) in elderly women. They analyzed 19,787 women with stage I or II breast cancer who received mastectomy as definitive surgery during 1991 to 1999. Multivariate logistic regression was used to investigate the association of distance with receipt of PMRT. They found that increasing distance to the nearest radiation treatment facility was independently associated with a decreased likelihood of receiving PMRT. Further analysis of these data indicated that the decline in PMRT use appeared at distances of more than 25 miles and was statistically significant when compared to patients living less than 25 miles from the radiation facility. For those patients living more than 75 miles from the nearest radiation facility, these effects appeared to be even more pronounced with people older than 75 years. These researchers stated that policymakers should consider these facts in resource allocation decisions about radiation treatment centers.[68]

Basu et al. analyzed hospital discharge data (HCUP), comparing severity thresholds between minorities and whites.[69] Using logistic models, they compared the association of distant admission with severity corresponding to each local threshold level, race, and type of hospital admission. The study used four discrete distance thresholds and examined how the severity thresholds for distance traveled for different types of admission might clarify different sources of disparities in health care utilization. The results indicated that minorities are more likely to have higher severity thresholds than whites in seeking distant hospital care, although these conclusions depended on the type of severity condition. The researchers suggested that if costly elective services were regionalized with appropriate outreach programs, then these disparities could be reduced.[69]

In another context, Higgs and White used GIS to analyze accessibility to services by different socioeconomic groups in England.[57] Kendal et al. suggested that the location strategy of collocation with facilities that provide complementary health services should be considered in efforts to improve accessibility to health care.[70] The Veterans Affairs (VA) health care system has been studied to determine the effects of proximity to services on their utilization.[71] LaVela et al. found that inpatient utilization decreased when travel distance to VA facilities increased for patients with some identified health problems.[72]

Problems experienced by patients in obtaining transportation to health facilities have become an issue in cancer prevention and control.[41,73] It is clear that travel distance can be a considerable burden to cancer patients seeking treatment. Results from many studies have led to efforts to model the location of mammography screening facilities in relation to their accessibility to different social and economic groups.[74]

11.7 CONCLUSIONS

Special issues arise when using geocodes to make and use distance estimates from people to facilities. The methods are changing fast as applications increasingly use GIS software and geospatial data to implement approaches. There are few standards to guide the appropriate use of the distances created by different systems. Although there have been many studies of geocoding issues, including the accuracy of geocoding procedures, the incompleteness of geocodes in typical application contexts, and the availability of masking methods to preserve privacy,[75] there have been few studies of comparable issues in estimating distances. Just as geocodes must be selected with care to match the intended purpose of their use, so must distance estimates be selected with care. Distance estimates, moreover, are notoriously sensitive to the geocoding completeness and accuracy of the facilities with which they are measured. It is not an exaggeration to state that if any one of the radiation therapy sites in a typical state is incorrectly geocoded or missing from the geocoding process, then the set of distances or potential distances of people to their closest facility are severely compromised. Caveat emptor should be prominent in the minds of users of such products of the geocoding process.

This said, there is no reverting to the archaic geographic accessibility measures used in health applications in the pre-GIS period. Taking arbitrary areas and expressing ratios of people per facility is by now an abandoned approach. The world people live in is one of residences, facilities, neighborhoods, places, and structures, all existing in a matrix of space and time. Many cancer prevention and control activities occur in this world, and their efficacy will increasingly be seen to depend on how well they work in it. The geocoding revolution is an essential foundation for planning and action for these activities.

REFERENCES

1. Rushton, G. Methods to evaluate geographic access to health services. *Journal of Public Health Management Practice,* 5(2), 93–100, 1999.
2. Love, D.; Lindquist, P. The geographical accessibility of hospitals to the aged: a geographic information systems analysis within Illinois. *Health Services Research,* 29, 629–651, 1995.
3. Martin, D.; Williams, H. Market-area analysis and accessibility to primary health-care centers. *Environment and Planning A,* 24, 1009–1019, 1992.
4. Williams, A. P.; Schwartz, W. B.; Newhouse, J. P.; Bennett, B. W. How many miles to the doctor? *New England Journal of Medicine,* 309, 958–963, 1983.
5. Love, R. F.; Morris, J. G.; Wesolowsky, G. O. *Facilities Location: Models and Methods.* North-Holland, Amsterdam, 1988.
6. Phibbs, C. S.; Luft, H. S. Correlation of travel time on roads versus straight line distance. *Medical Care Research and Review,* 52, 532–542, 1995.
7. Broome, F. R.; Meixler, D. B. The TIGER data base structure. *Cartography and Geographic Information Systems,* 17, 39–47, 1990.
8. Mapping Science Committee. *A Data Foundation for the National Spatial Data Infrastructure.* National Academy Press, Washington, DC, 1995.
9. World Health Organization. The signature domain and geographic coordinates: a standardized approach for uniquely identifying a health facility. In *Health Facility Assessment Technical Working Group,* WP-07–91, Carolina Population Center, University of North Carolina at Chapel Hill, 1–26, 2007.
10. Current, J. R.; Schilling, D. A. Elimination of source A and B errors in p-median location problems. *Geographical Analysis,* 19, 95, 1987.
11. Current, J. R.; Schilling, D. A. Analysis of errors due to demand data aggregation in the set covering and maximal covering location problems. *Geographical Analysis,* 22, 116–126, 1990.
12. Hillsman, E. L.; Rhoda, R. Errors in measuring distances from populations to service centers. *The Annals of Regional Science,* 12, 74–88, 1978.
13. Francis, R. L.; Lowe, T. J.; Rushton, G.; Rayco, M. B. A synthesis of aggregation methods for multi-facility location problems: strategies for containing error. *Geographical Analysis,* 31, 67–87, 1999.

14. Hewko, J.; Smoyer-Tomic, K. E.; Hodgson, M. J. Measuring neighborhood spatial accessibility to urban amenities: does aggregation error matter. *Environment and Planning A,* 34, 1185–1206, 2002.

15. Bhaduri, B.; Bright, E.; Coleman, P.; Dobson, J. LandScan: locating people is what matters. *Geoinformatics,* 5(2) 34–37, 2002.

16. Bracken, I.; Martin, D. The generation of spatial population distributions from census centroid data. *Environmental Planning A,* 21, 537–543, 1989.

17. Fortney, J.; Rost, K.; Warren, J. Comparing alternative methods of measuring geographic access to health services. *Health Services and Outcomes Research Methodology,* 1, 173–184, 2000.

18. Rushton, G. Use of location-allocation models for improving the geographical accessibility of rural services in developing countries. *International Regional Science Review,* 9, 217–240, 1984.

19. Densham, P. J. Spatial decision support systems. In *Geographical Information Systems: Principles and Applications*, Maguire, D. J.; Goodchild, M. F.; Rhind, D. W., Eds. Longman (copublished by Wiley), New York, 1991, pp. 403–412.

20. Gorr, W.; Johnson, M.; Roehrig, S. Spatial decision support system for home-delivered services. *Journal of Geographical Systems,* 3, 181–197, 2001.

21. Rushton, G., Spatial decision support systems. In *International Encyclopedia of the Social and Behavioral Sciences*, Smelser, N. J.; Baltes, P. B., Eds. Pergamon, Oxford, UK, 2001, Vol. 22, p. 14785–14788.

22. Wong, D. W. S.; Meyer, J. W. A spatial decision support system approach to evaluate the efficiency of a Meals-on-Wheels program. *The Professional Geographer,* 45, 332–341, 1993.

23. Walsh, S. J.; Page, P. H.; Gesler, W. M. Normative models and healthcare planning: network-based simulations within a geographic information system environment. *Health Services Research,* 32, 243–260, 1997.

24. Ayeni, B.; Rushton, G.; McNulty, M. L. Improving the geographical accessibility of health care in rural areas: a Nigerian case study. *Social Science and Medicine,* 25, 1083–1094, 1987.

25. Cromley, E. K.; McLafferty, S. *GIS and Public Health*. Guilford Press, New York, 2002.

26. Cromley, E. K.; Shannon, G. W. Locating ambulatory medical care facilities for the elderly. *Health Services Research,* 21, 499–514, 1986.

27. McLafferty, S. L. GIS and health care. *Annual Review of Public Health,* 24, 25, 2003.

28. Liu, S.; Zhu, X. An integrated GIS approach to accessibility analysis. *Transactions in GIS,* 8, 45–62, 2004.

29. McGuirk, M. A.; Porell, F. W. Spatial patterns of hospital utilization: the impact of distance and time. *Inquiry,* 21, 84–95, 1984.

30. van Eck, J. R. R.; de Jong, T. Accessibility analysis and spatial competition effects in the context of GIS-supported service location planning. *Computers, Environment and Urban Systems,* 23, 75–89, 1999.

31. Fotheringham, A. S.; O'Kelly, M. E. *Spatial Interaction Models: Formulations and Applications*. Kluwer Academic, Dordrecht, Netherlands, 1989.

32. Geertman, S. C. M.; Eck, J. R. R. GIS and models of accessibility potential: an application in planning. *International Journal of Geographical Information Systems,* 9, 67–80, 1995.

33. Lovett, A.; Haynes, R.; Sunnenberg, G.; Gale, S. Car travel time and accessibility by bus to general practitioner services: a study using patient registers and GIS. *Social Science and Medicine,* 55, 97–111, 2002.

34. Weber, J.; Kwan, M. P. Bringing time back in: a study on the influence of travel time variations and facility opening hours on individual accessibility. *The Professional Geographer,* 54, 226–240, 2002.

35. Guagliardo, M. F. Spatial accessibility of primary care: concepts, methods and challenges. *International Journal of Health Geographics,* 3: 3, 2004.
36. Miller, H. J. Modelling accessibility using space-time prism concepts within geographical information systems. *International Journal of Geographical Information Systems,* 5, 287–301, 1991.
37. Miller, H. J. Measuring space-time accessibility benefits within transportation networks: basic theory and computational procedures. *Geographical Analysis,* 31, 1–26, 1999.
38. Kwan, M. P. Space-time and integral measures of individual accessibility: a comparative analysis using a point-based framework. *Geographical Analysis,* 30, 191–216, 1998.
39. Kwan, M. P.; Janelle, D. G.; Goodchild, M. F. Accessibility in space and time: a theme in spatially integrated social science. *Journal of Geographical Systems,* 5, 1–3, 2003.
40. Kwan, M. P.; Murray, A. T.; O'Kelly, M. E.; Tiefelsdorf, M. Recent advances in accessibility research: representation, methodology and applications. *Journal of Geographical Systems,* 5, 129–138, 2003.
41. Payne, S.; Jarrett, N.; Jeffs, D. The impact of travel on cancer patients' experiences of treatment: a literature review. *European Journal of Cancer Care (England),* 9, 197–203, 2000.
42. Horner, M. W. Exploring metropolitan accessibility and urban structure. *Urban Geography,* 25, 264–284, 2004.
43. Talen, E.; Anselin, L. Assessing spatial equity: an evaluation of measures of accessibility to public playgrounds. *Environment and Planning A,* 30, 593–613, 1998.
44. Armstrong, M. P.; Densham, P. J.; Lolonis, P.; Rushton, G. Cartographic displays to support locational decision making. *Cartography and Geographic Information Systems,* 19, 154–164, 1992.
45. National Cancer Institute cancer mortality maps and graphs Web site. http://www3. cancer.gov/atlasplus/
46. Richards, T. B.; Croner, C. M.; Rushton, G.; Brown, C. K.; Fowler, L. Geographic information systems and public health: mapping the future. *Public Health Reports,* 114, 359–373, 1999.
47. Ballas, L. K.; Elkin, E. B.; Schrag, D.; Minsky, B. D.; Bach, P. B. Radiation therapy facilities in the United States. *International Journal of Radiation Oncology, Biology, Physics,* 66, 1204–1211, 2006.
48. Lin, S. J., Access to community pharmacies by the elderly in Illinois: a geographic information systems analysis. *Journal of Medical Systems,* 28, 301–309, 2004.
49. Clark, W.; Rushton, G. A method for analyzing the relationship of a population to distributed facilities. *Environment and Behavior,* 2, 192–207, 1970.
50. Brainard, J. S.; Lovett, A. A.; Bateman, I. J. Using isochrone surfaces in travel-cost models. *Journal of Transport Geography,* 5, 117–126, 1997.
51. Lee, R. C. Current approaches to shortage area designation. *Journal of Rural Health,* 7, 437–450, 1991.
52. Guagliardo, M. F.; Ronzio, C. R.; Cheung, I.; Chacko, E.; Joseph, J. G. Physician accessibility: an urban case study of pediatric providers. *Health and Place,* 10, 273–283, 2004.
53. Luo, W. Using a GIS-based floating catchment method to assess areas with shortage of physicians. *Health and Place,* 10, 1–11, 2004.
54. Luo, W.; Wang, F. Measures of spatial accessibility to health care in a GIS environment: synthesis and a case study in the Chicago region. *Environment and Planning B,* 30, 865–884, 2003.
55. Rushton, G.; Peleg, I.; Banerjee, A.; Smith, G.; West, M. Analyzing geographic patterns of disease incidence: rates of late-stage colorectal cancer in Iowa. *Journal of Medical Systems,* 28, 223–236, 2004.
56. Weber, J.; Kwan, M. P. Evaluating the effects of geographic contexts on individual accessibility: a multilevel approach. *Urban Geography,* 24, 647–671, 2003.

57. Higgs, G.; White, S. D. Changes in service provision in rural areas. Part 1: the use of GIS in analysing accessibility to services in rural deprivation research. *Journal of Rural Studies,* 13, 441–450, 1997.

58. Shannon, G. W.; Bashshur, R. L.; Metzner, C. A. The concept of distance as a factor in accessijility and utilization of health care. *Medical Care Review,* 26, 143–161, 1969.

59. Weiss, J. E. Determinants of medical care utilization: the impact of spatial factors. *Inquiry,* 8, 50–57, 1971.

60. Ricketts, T. C.; Savitz, L. Access to health services. In *Geographic Methods for Health Services Research.* Eds. Ricketts, T.C., Savitz, L.A., Gessler, W.M., and Osborne, D.N. University Press of America, Lanham, MD, 1994, pp. 91–112.

61. Fortney, J.; Rost, K.; Zhang, M.; Warren, J. The impact of geographic accessibility on the intensity and quality of depression treatment. *Medical Care,* 37, 884–893, 1999.

62. Joseph, A. E.; Phillips, D. R. *Accessibility and Utilization: Geographical Perspectives on Health Care Delivery.* Harper and Row, New York, 1984.

63. Voti, L.; Richardson, L. C.; Reis, I. M.; Fleming, L. E.; MacKinnon, J.; Coebergh, J. W. Treatment of local breast carcinoma in Florida. *Cancer,* 106, 201–207, 2006.

64. Celaya, M. O.; Rees, J. R.; Gibson, J. J.; Riddle, B. L.; Greenberg, E. R. Travel distance and season of diagnosis affect treatment choices for women with early-stage breast cancer in a predominantly rural population (United States). *Cancer Causes and Control,* 17, 851–856, 2006.

65. Nattinger, A. B.; Kneusel, R. T.; Hoffmann, R. G.; Gilligan, M. A. Relationship of distance from a radiotherapy facility and initial breast cancer treatment. *Journal of the National Cancer Institute,* 93, 1344–1346, 2001.

66. Rushton, G.; West, M. Women with localized breast cancer selecting mastectomy treatment, Iowa, 1991–1996. *Public Health Reports,* 114, 370–371, 1999.

67. Athas, W. F.; Adams-Cameron, M.; Hunt, W. C.; Amir-Fazli, A.; Key, C. R. Travel distance to radiation therapy and receipt of radiotherapy following breast-conserving surgery. *Journal of the National Cancer Institute,* 92, 269–271, 2000.

68. Punglia, R. S.; Weeks, J. C.; Neville, B. A.; Earle, C. C. Effect of distance to radiation treatment facility on use of radiation therapy after mastectomy in elderly women. *International Journal of Radiation Oncology, Biology, Physics,* 66, 56–63, 2006.

69. Basu, J., Friedman, B., and Burstin, H. Preventable hospitalization and medicaid managed care: Does race matler? *Journal of Health Care for the Poor and Underserved,* 17(1), 101–115, 2006.

70. Kendal, A. P.; Peterson, A.; Manning, C.; Xu, F.; Neville, L. J.; Hogue, C. Improving the health of infants on Medicaid by collocating special supplemental nutrition clinics with managed care provider sites. *American Journal of Public Health,* 92, 399–403, 2002.

71. Burgess, J. F., Jr.; DeFiore, D. A. The effect of distance to VA facilities on the choice and level of utilization of VA outpatient services. *Social Science and Medicine,* 39, 95–104, 1994.

72. LaVela, S. L.; Smith, B.; Weaver, F. M.; Miskevics, S. A. Geographical proximity and health care utilization in veterans with SCI&D in the USA. *Social Science and Medicine,* 59, 2387–2399, 2004.

73. Guidry, J. J.; Aday, L. A.; Zhang, D.; Winn, R. J. Transportation as a barrier to cancer treatment. *Cancer Practice,* 5, 361–366, 1997.

74. Hyndman, J. C.; Holman, C. D. Differential effects on socioeconomic groups of modelling the location of mammography screening clinics using geographic information systems. *Australia and New Zealand Journal of Public Health,* 24, 281–286, 2000.

75. Rushton, G.; Armstrong, M. P.; Gittler, J.; Greene, B. R.; Pavlik, C. E.; West, M. M.; Zimmerman, D. L. Geocoding in cancer research: a review. *American Journal of Preventive Medicine,* 30, S16–S24, 2006.

12 Cancer Registry Data and Geocoding
Privacy, Confidentiality, and Security Issues

Josephine Gittler

CONTENTS

12.1 INTRODUCTION

Central population-based cancer registries have been established in all 50 states of the United States and in the District of Columbia.[1,2] State public health agencies usually administer these registries, but they sometimes contract with, or otherwise authorize, other entities to be responsible for registry administration. To reduce the burden of cancer through cancer prevention and control, these registries carry out the public health function of cancer surveillance: "The ongoing, timely and systematic collection and analysis of information on cancer risk factors ..., screening and early detection, new cancer cases, cancer deaths, and extent of disease at diagnosis, treatment, clinical management, and survival."[3 at p. 7]

Cancer registries are increasingly applying geographic information system (GIS) technology to their cancer data.[4] According to the World Health Organization, a GIS is "a computer-aided database management and map technology that organizes and stores large amounts of multi-purpose information" and "adds the dimension of geographic analysis to information technology (IT) by providing an interface between the data and a map."[5] Registries can use GIS technology to geocode their cancer data, which entails assigning geographic identifiers (geocodes) to computer records of cancer cases and cancer deaths, thereby tying the information in these records to a geographic location or space.[6] Geocoding permits the creation of visual representations of geographic patterns of cancer incidence and mortality rates in maps.[6] By linking geocoded cancer data sets to other geocoded data sets, including demographic, socioeconomic, environmental, and health services data sets, it also becomes possible to identify and analyze relationships between cancer cases and deaths and a number of other variables.[6]

Health facilities and health care practitioners are legally mandated to report information about cancer cases to central population-based registries.[7] Under mandatory reporting laws, health care providers do not have to obtain the consent of cancer patients for the reporting of information about their cases.[7] The reportable information is personal health information, which means it "relates to the health status or condition of an individual and the provision of health care to an individual."[8 at 45 CFR § 160.103] The reportable information also is individually identifiable, which means it "identifies the individual" who is the subject of the information, or "there is a reasonable basis to believe ... [it] can be used to identify the individual."[8 at 45 CFR § 160.103]

The goal of this chapter is to provide an overview of privacy and confidentiality issues arising from the reporting of cases to central cancer registries and the use and disclosure of geocoded registry data and other registry data. This chapter also addresses the issue of ensuring the security of cancer registry data before, during, and after geocoding. These issues have significant public policy and legal implications.

12.2 BACKGROUND

12.2.1 INFORMATION PRIVACY: DEFINITIONS AND CONCEPTS

The privacy of the personal health information of cancer patients reported to cancer registries falls within the larger category of what is known as information privacy. There is no single accepted definition of information privacy and other forms of privacy. Privacy means many different things to different people, and its meaning varies in different contexts and different settings and has evolved over time.[9–14]

Although a detailed discussion of the meanings ascribed to privacy, particularly information privacy, is beyond the scope of this chapter, a prominent privacy scholar, Randall Bezanson, has identified several core concepts of information privacy that appear frequently in the privacy literature. He described five distinct but overlapping concepts that are directly relevant to the privacy of personal health information reported to cancer registries and the confidentiality of the information once reported.[9]

The first privacy concept, which Bezanson described, involves protection of an individual from "public disclosure of embarrassing, intimate, or personal information" and "against a loss of ... dignity in the community stemming from personal feelings of ostracization and embarrassment and psychological harm that often follows from knowledge that others know our true secrets."[9 at p. 7] The second concept involves protection of an individual's "ability to maintain secrecy or control disclosure of information in the interest of shaping or maintaining ... public and private identity and in the interest of protecting relationships with others, whether personal, intimate, professional, or public."[9 at p. 7] The third concept involves protection of an individual "against concrete economic or social harm that may flow from disclosure of information about oneself by others."[9 at p. 8] The fourth concept involves protection "against harm from disclosure to other persons."[9 at p. 8]

All four of these concepts have in common a focus on the disclosure of personal information that the individual, who is the subject of the information, does not wish to be disclosed, and that is individually identifiable. These concepts also contemplate a variety of psychological, social and economic harms and negative consequences flowing from such disclosure.[15,16] Some kind of harm or negative consequence is particularly likely to flow from the nonconsensual disclosure of individually identifiable personal health information due to its often sensitive and detailed nature. Thus, it is not unusual for an individual's medical record, a primary source of personal health information, to have both objective and subjective information pertaining to physical health, mental health, behavior and lifestyle, such as sexual practices and substance use and abuse, information pertaining to family status and history and relationships with others, financial infromation, such as employment and income level, and demographic information.[15,16]

Bezanson described a fifth privacy concept involving "control or ownership of information about oneself ... whether the information is personal and intimate or not and whether the disclosure is made or not."[9 at p. 8] He explained that this concept "concerns an individual's autonomy — the power to protect individuality — which is manifested in the individual's ownership and control over disclosures [of personal information] as well as the power to restrict later uses and disclosures by others."[9 at p. 9] It follows from this privacy concept that the use and disclosure of an individual's personal information without the individual's consent in and of itself can constitute a privacy violation.

12.2.2 PRIVACY OF PERSONAL HEALTH INFORMATION

Most Americans consider personal health information, like that reported to cancer registries, to be highly private information.[17–23] For example, a national public opinion poll conducted in 2000 by the Gallup Organization found that poll respondents rated personal health information and personal financial information as the two most sensitive types of personal information; the poll further found that 92% of respondents felt it was very important or somewhat important for medical records to be kept confidential.[20]

The general public appears to associate the privacy of personal health information with its control, and there is widespread opposition among members of the general public to allowing access to their personal health information without their consent.[17,18,20] The 2000 Gallup poll is illustrative. Of the poll respondents, 71% opposed permitting local and state health departments nonconsensual access to their medical records; and 67% opposed permitting medical researchers nonconsensual access.[20] A later National Consumer Health Survey, conducted in 2005 by Forrester Research for the California Healthcare Foundation, reported somewhat similar results. Only 20% of respondents were willing to share their personal health information with government agencies, and only 42% felt that researchers had a right to use this information.[17]

Health professionals also regard the privacy of personal health information as important. As far back as the fourth century BC, physicians taking the Hippocratic oath swore to keep secret what their patients divulged to them in the course of the physician-patient relationship.[12,24,25] Today, it is well established that the confidentiality of patient communications is an essential component of trusting physician-patient relationships and trusting relationships between other health professionals and their patients because the assurance of confidentiality encourages patients to share fully the information that is a prerequisite for appropriate diagnosis and treatment.[12,24,26–29]

The advent of the information age, marked by the creation of information infrastructures comprised of computers, electronic databases, the Internet, and other information technologies, has intensified long-standing concerns about information privacy,[17,30–38] and the growth in the use of information technologies in the health care system has generated special concerns about the confidentiality of personal health information in medical records and health care databases.[16,24,28,29,39–45] As a result of dramatic advances in information technologies, vast amounts of personal information, including personal health information, are now electronically collected, managed, stored, and analyzed; huge electronic databases containing personal information have been established in both the public and private sectors; and electronic records are easily and almost instantaneously transmitted to multiple sites worldwide. Many privacy experts and advocates view the proliferation of electronic records and databases as posing a privacy threat because they are susceptible to use in ways that compromise the privacy of the information they contain. Although GIS, geocoding, and associated technologies have attracted relatively little attention from privacy experts and advocates, some authorities on GIS and geocoding have recognized that their use may lead to privacy violations,[6,46–62] and a few of these authorities specifically have recognized that the application of GIS technology to cancer registry data may lead to privacy violations.[4,6]

In the last decade, public opinion polls have repeatedly revealed that health care consumers are apprehensive about the privacy of their personal health information, especially information in their medical records.[17–19, 21, 23, 29, 63, 64] The 2005 National Consumer Health Privacy Survey found that 67% of respondents were "very concerned" or "somewhat concerned" about the privacy of their medical records.[17] Public opinion polls indicate that consumers are especially apprehensive about the impact of the trend toward electronic medical records on the confidentiality and security of those records.[17–19,21,23,29,64] A 2005

Harris Interactive national public opinion poll found that 69% of respondents were very concerned or somewhat concerned that a national electronic record system would lead to more sharing of their medical records without their knowledge, and 70% were very concerned or somewhat concerned that information in their medical records might be leaked because of security breaches.[23,64]

Lack of confidence in the adequacy of privacy protections may lead to "privacy-protective" behaviors on the part of health care consumers. To prevent others from finding out about their health status and health care, health care consumers may give incomplete or inaccurate information to their physician and other health care providers; they may ask their physician to conceal their diagnosis by recording a less-serious or less-embarrassing diagnosis than the actual diagnosis or by not recording the actual diagnosis at all; they may pay claims for health services themselves without submitting them to insurers; they may go to physicians other than their regular physician for certain types of health problems and services; they may avoid diagnostic tests and procedures; and they may delay or even forgo care altogether.[17,18,28,29,63]

The 2005 National Consumer Health Survey indicated that 15% of respondents had engaged in at least one privacy-protective behavior; respondents diagnosed with a disease were the most likely to have engaged in these behaviors, and 11% of respondents with cancer had engaged in these behaviors.[17] Although the immediate consequence of privacy-protective behaviors is that people may not receive appropriate health care, such behaviors also may undermine efforts of entities, like cancer registries, to collect complete and accurate data for public health and research purposes.[22,63]

12.2.3 LEGAL PROTECTIONS OF PERSONAL HEALTH INFORMATION PRIVACY

Legal protections have been afforded, to some degree, to information privacy, including personal health information privacy. Information privacy law is composed of a large, complicated, and confusing array of federal and state constitutional provisions, statutes, administrative regulations, and judicial decisions.[12,14,65]

Historically, legal privacy protections have been a matter of state law. Responding to increasing concerns about the privacy of personal health information, in the 1970s states began to enact privacy protection legislation applicable to patient health records.[66] States usually have at least several different statutes that deal with the privacy and confidentiality of patient health records and that vary in the scope and the level of protection they provide.[66–68] These state statutes and their accompanying administrative regulations form a diverse and inconsistent collection of legal protections for the privacy of personal health information.[66–68]

The historic role of the states as the predominant source of legal protections for personal health information privacy was altered when the U.S. Department of Health and Human Services (HHS) issued federal regulations, known as the Privacy Rule, pursuant to the Health Insurance Portability and Accountability Act of 1996 (HIPAA).[69] The Privacy Rule, which became effective in 2003, established for the first time national standards for protection of the privacy of personal health information.[8] In addition, various federal statutes and administrative regulations have information privacy requirements with which federal agencies and federally funded and regulated research projects that collect and hold personal health information must comply.[54,58,70]

There is a consensus both that personal health information is deserving of legal protection from unwarranted invasion and infringement and that this information is not entitled to absolute privacy protection.[10] As a result, laws protecting the privacy of personal health information tend to reflect not only the interests of individuals in the privacy of information about their health status and health care but also the interests of society in the acquisition and utilization of this information to improve public health.[29,39–41,71]

12.3 REPORTING OF CANCER CASES TO CANCER REGISTRIES

12.3.1 The Existing Legal Framework for Reporting

The reporting of information about cases of cancer patients by health care facilities and practitioners to population-based central cancer registries raises privacy concerns. To understand privacy issues related to cancer case reporting, it is first necessary to understand the legal framework within which reporting takes place.

12.3.1.1 HIPAA Privacy Rule

The reporting of cancer cases to cancer registries is controlled in the first instance by the HIPAA Privacy Rule.[8] The Rule sets a floor — not a ceiling — for privacy protections. Accordingly, the Rule preempts contrary state laws, but state laws that have more stringent privacy protections than the Rule continue in effect.[8 at 45 CFR §§ 160.202-203]

In general, the Privacy Rule prohibits covered entities from disclosing an individual's protected health information (PHI) without written authorization of the individual who is the subject of the information (individual authorization) except for certain designated purposes under certain designated circumstances. The individual authorization requirement is intended to ensure that covered entities obtain a patient's informed consent in writing before disclosing PHI.

PHI is health information that is individually identifiable and is held or transmitted in any form or medium (electronic, written, or oral) by a covered entity.[8 at 45 CFR § 164.501] Hence, information about cancer cases, containing individually identifiable information that a covered entity reports to a cancer registry, is PHI under the Privacy Rule.

Covered entities include health care providers, health plans, and health clearinghouses. Health care providers are any persons or entities furnishing, billing, or paying for health care.[8 at 45 CFR §§ 160.102–103] Hence, health practitioners and health facilities providing diagnostic and treatment services to cancer patients are covered entities within the meaning of the Privacy Rule. Because cancer registries are not covered entities under the Rule, they are not subject to the Rule's provisions. But, health care providers (i.e., covered entities), in making reports about cancer cases (i.e., PHI) to registries, must comply with the Rule's provisions limiting the use and disclosure of PHI.

The Privacy Rule enumerates exceptions to the prohibition of PHI disclosure without individual authorization applicable to the reporting of information about cancer cases to cancer registries. One provision of the Rule permits a covered entity to disclose PHI without individual authorization to the extent disclosure "is required by law."[8 at 45 CFR § 164.512(a)] Another provision of the Rule permits a covered entity to disclose PHI without individual authorization to "a public health authority that is authorized by law to collect or receive such information for purposes of preventing or controlling disease ... including but not limited to, reporting of disease ... and the conduct of public health surveillance, public health investigations and public health interventions."[8 at 45 CFR § 164.512(b)] Public health authority is defined to encompass both the state public health agencies and the other entities, acting under a grant of authority from these agencies, which administer cancer registries.[8 at 45 CFR § 164.502]

These provisions of the Privacy Rule can be criticized as unduly broad and open ended. They also can be criticized on the ground that they are inconsistent with the Rule's objective of providing uniform minimum standards that protect the privacy of personal health information. Regardless of these criticisms, the Rule clearly allows health practitioners and facilities to report individually identifiable information about cancer cases to a cancer registry without individual authorization pursuant to state laws requiring or authorizing such reporting.[72,73]

12.3.1.2 State Laws

Although the Privacy Rule permits the mandatory reporting of individually identifiable information about cancer cases to cancer registries, it is left to states to determine whether actually to mandate reporting. At the present time, 50 states and the District of Columbia have cancer reporting laws made up of a variety of statutes and their accompanying administrative regulations.[7] In some states, statutes specifically provide for the mandatory reporting of cancer cases. In other states, statutes provide general authorization for the mandatory reporting of cases of diseases as specified by the state public health agency in administrative regulations. See the appendix following chapter 13 for a state-by-state listing of state statutes and administrative regulations dealing with reporting of cancer cases.

All of the existing cancer reporting laws call for mandatory reporting of cancer cases.[7] They also typically require that cancer case reports include individual identifiers (e.g., name, address, date of birth, social security number, etc.) together with other demographic information and information about the cancer diagnosis and treatment.[7]

It should be noted that the Cancer Registries Amendment Act, federal legislation enacted in 1992, makes federal financial assistance available to states to support population-based statewide cancer registries.[74] To receive this assistance, a state must have a state law requiring reporting of cancer cases to a statewide registry.[74]

12.3.2 RATIONALE FOR MANDATORY REPORTING AND REPORTING OF INDIVIDUALLY IDENTIFIABLE INFORMATION

Given the previously described privacy concepts, existing state laws mandating reporting of the personal health information of cancer patients without their consent are problematic from a privacy standpoint. State laws mandating reporting of individually identifiable information are even more problematic, especially if disclosure of the information may prove harmful.

Because requiring reporting of the individually identifiable health information of cancer patients without their consent poses privacy problems, the state laws requiring such reporting would seem to deserve close scrutiny from public policymakers. Nevertheless, it appears these laws have been adopted without much discussion.

State cancer reporting statutes and administrative regulations are the outgrowth of a broader effort to make certain that public health authorities are notified of actual and potential public health problems. Health care providers are legally obligated to report not only cancers but also other diseases and conditions to public health authorities.[40,75] Although the legally mandated reporting of individually identifiable information about some diseases and conditions — the most recent example is HIV/AIDS (human immunodeficiency virus/acquired immunodeficiency syndrome) — have generated controversy, mandatory cancer reporting laws have not proved controversial.[75,76]

The United Kingdom, unlike the United States, has witnessed a heated debate over whether patients should be legally required to give their explicit informed consent before health care providers can transmit their identifiable health information to disease registries and medical researchers.[77,78] The U.K. cancer registries and their supporters have strenuously opposed a patient consent requirement for reporting of cancer cases to registries, asserting that it would hinder efforts of registries to collect data about cancer cases and could even bring about their collapse.[79–82]

The basic rationale for mandatory cancer reporting is to ensure the completeness and accuracy of registry data in order to ensure the effectiveness of cancer surveillance.[81–83] This rationale rests on the premise that a requirement of informed patient consent for reporting of cancer cases to registries would produce a decline in reporting, and that a decline in cancer case reporting would undermine the ability of registries to collect complete and accurate data.[79–83] It also rests on the premise that the patients who select to participate might not be representative of the cancer population as a whole or segments thereof, which would introduce selection bias into cancer registry data.[84–86] In addition, it is contended that obtaining the consent of cancer patients would prove costly, time consuming, logistically unworkable, and unduly burdensome for already overburdened health care providers and registries.[83]

There is some empirical evidence indicating that an opt-in consent model under which a patient must expressly consent to reporting would lead to a reduction in cancer case reporting and selection bias in registry data.[77,78,87–91] In predicting the effect of a patient consent requirement on the collection of data by registries, it is important to distinguish between the opt-in consent model and the opt-out consent model under which consent is presumed unless patients affirmatively make known their refusal to consent. The opt-out model is associated with considerably lower patient refusal rates than the opt-in model.[84,85,92–94] Therefore, it would seem that the opt-out model would be less likely, perhaps far less likely, to impair the data collection efforts of registries than the opt-in model. A priority for future research and demonstration projects should be the use of different models of consent with respect to the reporting of cancers and a comparison of their impact on reporting rates.

The rationale for reporting individually identifiable information, rather than anonymized or deidentified data, is similar to the rationale for mandatory reporting, namely, to ensure the completeness and accuracy of registry data.[72,77,95] The inclusion of individual identifiers in reports of cancer cases enables registries to link reports about the same patient to avoid duplicate counting of cases.[72,95] It also enables registries to link their cancer case reports with data from different sources to conduct patient follow-up and other surveillance activities.[95] The inclusion of individual geographic identifiers, such as addresses of cancer patients, in reports of cancer cases is necessary for geocoding of registry data and its linkage with other geocoded data sets.

12.3.3 JUSTIFICATIONS FOR REPORTING REQUIREMENTS

Even if state laws mandating the reporting of individually identifiable information about cancer cases to cancer registries are necessary to ensure the completeness and accuracy of registry data, it is not self-evident that this should be regarded as adequate justification for these laws. Because data collection is not an end in itself, it remains to be considered whether the costs of these reporting laws in terms of their effect on the privacy interests of cancer patients is justified by its public health benefits that translate into societal benefits.

12.3.3.1 Privacy Costs

A precise assessment of the privacy costs of existing state cancer reporting laws is difficult because of several factors. One factor is that privacy violations form a continuum ranging from the serious to the inconsequential.[96] Another factor is that the assessment of whether privacy has been compromised and how much it has been compromised is highly subjective, differing from person to person, and is influenced by the situation and the context in which it occurs.[96]

One source of data relevant to an assessment of privacy costs is the previously described national public opinion polls. As it has been pointed out, extensive polling data have documented the attitudes of the American public toward the privacy of personal health information for a considerable period of time. According to these polls, large majorities of poll respondents consistently have attached a great deal of importance to personal health information privacy. Large majorities consistently have opposed allowing access to their personal health information without their consent — an opposition that extends to nonconsensual access by public health agencies, medical researchers, and other researchers. Large majorities consistently have reported that they do not have confidence in the adequacy of privacy, confidentiality, and security protections, which may lead to privacy-protective behaviors by health care consumers, including cancer patients. These polling data suggest that the American public, as well as individual cancer patients, may have objections to legally requiring reporting of identifiable cancer patient information without patient consent.

Yet, the national public opinion polling data about the public's attitudes toward the privacy of personal health information does not necessarily dictate the conclusion that existing state cancer reporting laws may lack the support of the general public and cancer patients because of privacy concerns. Interestingly, a 2006 study conducted in the United Kingdom found that the majority of study participants did not object to the transfer of identifiable patient information without patient consent to the National Cancer Registry.[84] A factor that may have influenced the results of this study was that respondents were told that reports made to the registry would be confidential, and that they would be used for public health purposes.[84] One can only speculate whether replication of this study in the United States would produce similar results. Another priority for future research should be the perceptions of the public and of cancer patients regarding the privacy, confidentiality, and security of patient-specific information about cancer cases, their perceptions regarding the acceptability of nonconsensual reporting of such information to cancer registries, and the variables that influence these perceptions.

Finally, it should be noted that advocates for laws requiring health care providers to report individually identifiable personal health information take somewhat inconsistent positions regarding the privacy implications of these types of reporting requirements. On the one hand, they take the position that these laws affect patient privacy minimally even though the reporting of individually identifiable personal health information of patients takes place without their consent. On the other hand, they take the position that, if informed patient consent were required, then the data collection efforts of registries would suffer because a significant number of patients would refuse to consent to reporting for privacy reasons.

12.3.3.2 Public Health and Societal Benefits

A logical place to begin an assessment of the public health and societal benefits of existing state cancer reporting laws is with their historical antecedents in state and municipal laws compelling health care providers to notify local public health authorities of cases of communicable diseases. These laws were enacted in the late 19th and early 20th centuries when outbreaks and epidemics of these diseases were common and exacted a terrible toll in illness and death.[97] Communicable disease reporting laws produced the data needed for communicable disease surveillance systems that became the foundation for public health interventions to prevent and control the spread of these diseases.[98] These interventions were directed at detecting and eliminating the source of infectious disease outbreaks and epidemics, identifying and successfully treating people with infectious diseases, and preventing people from becoming infected with these diseases.[98]

Over the years, cancers were added to an ever-lengthening list of diseases and conditions reportable by law to public health authorities.[97] Because cancers are not contagious and cannot be transmitted from one person to another person, cancer patients do not pose the danger to the health of others that patients with communicable diseases pose. Therefore, the argument for mandatory cancer reporting laws can be seen as less compelling than the argument for mandatory communicable disease reporting laws.

Today, however, communicable diseases — with a few exceptions like HIV/AIDS — are no longer the threat they once were, and cancer has become a major cause of morbidity and mortality. In 2002, over 1.2 million Americans were diagnosed with cancer, and over 557,000 died of cancer, making it the nation's second leading cause of death.[99,100] The financial costs of cancer, as well as its human costs, are high. In 2005, the cost of providing health care to cancer patients and the costs of loss in productivity of cancer patients totaled an estimated \$210 billion.[99] In light of these costs, cancer now must be seen as an even greater public health problem than communicable diseases.

Reports of cancer cases to cancer registries are the primary source of data for cancer surveillance, and cancer registries are an integral and critical component of cancer surveillance systems.[1,2,100,101] Applications of GIS technology in public health activities, such as public health surveillance, are expanding rapidly,[4,5,102–108], and GIS technology can be used to geocode cancer registry data in conjunction with cancer surveillance.[4,6,109–111]

Because the purpose of state cancer reporting laws is to generate data for cancer surveillance, an assessment of the benefits of these laws must turn on an assessment of the benefits of cancer surveillance. The ultimate aim of cancer surveillance, based on data reported to registries, is to promote the development, implementation, and evaluation of strategies to reduce cancer morbidity and mortality.[2,100] In *Healthy People 2010*, the U.S. Department of Health and Human Services set forth a statement of health objectives for the nation, and *Healthy People 2010* declares that cancer registry surveillance data are "essential" for cancer prevention and control activities.[100 at pp. 3–27] It enunciates four main uses for surveillance data : (1) "advancing clinical, epidemiological and health services research" to "better understand and tackle the cancer burden"; (2) "planning and evaluating cancer control programs"; (3) "allocating preventative and treatment resources"; and (4) "responding to concerns from citizens about the occurrence of cancer in their communities."[100 at pp. 3–27]

GIS technology can substantially enhance the ability of cancer registries and public health agencies to carry out cancer surveillance.[1,5,109] GIS technology is used in cancer surveillance to determine and analyze the geographic distribution of cancers and trends over time and to determine and analyze populations at risk and risk factors.[1,5] GIS technology also can be of value in a variety of surveillance-related cancer prevention and control efforts.[1,4,5,109,112]

One of the best-known applications of GIS technology is in epidemiological research regarding the distribution and determinants of diseases and other health-related events in human populations.[113] Epidemiologists traditionally have mapped the location of cases of diseases to study the relationships among location, environment, and disease and to ascertain the etiology, or causes, of disease outbreaks and epidemics. During an 1854 cholera epidemic in London, Dr. John Snow, one of the founders of modern epidemiology, mapped the geographic location of cholera cases, which led him to conclude that the water supply from the infamous "Broad street pump" was the source of the epidemic.[114] The mapping capabilities of GIS technology make it an ideal and powerful tool for modern epidemiologic cancer research and other epidemiologic research.[4,5,115]

In summary, an assessment of the public health and societal benefits of state cancer reporting laws entails an assessment of the public health and societal benefits of cancer surveillance that these laws make possible. Although the potential benefits of surveillance, measured by its contribution to reducing the cancer burden, are undoubtedly great, it is not easy to quantify its actual benefits on the basis of readily available evidence.

The ultimate issue, of course, is whether these laws in their present form strike an appropriate balance between privacy interests and public health and societal interests. It is clear that the public health, GIS, and cancer research communities support such laws. It is less clear that, if asked for an opinion, members of the general public and cancer patients would support such laws. A prime determinant of the acceptability of these laws to the general public and to cancer patients may be whether the confidentiality of the information reported is adequately protected and whether its security is adequately safeguarded.

12.4 USE AND DISCLOSURE OF REGISTRY DATA

12.4.1 CONFIDENTIALITY: POLICIES, PRACTICES, AND LEGAL REQUIREMENTS

Just as the reporting of information about cases of cancer patients to cancer registries raises privacy concerns, its use and disclosure after it is reported raises privacy concerns. Given the private nature of this information, it is considered highly confidential. There is no single standard definition of either the term privacy or the term confidentiality. Although these terms are sometimes used interchangeably, they are not synonymous.[53,58,116] Privacy broadly defined is "an individual's claim to control the terms under which information ... is acquired, disclosed and used,"[117 at p. 2] whereas confidentiality broadly defined is "the assurance that information will be held in confidence with access limited to appropriate persons."[118 at p. 2]

12.4.1.1 Applicable Laws

The HIPAA Privacy Rule regulates the reporting of information about cancer cases to state cancer registries by health care providers. But, once the information is reported, the rule no longer applies because the rule is applicable only to covered entities, and cancer registries, unlike health care providers, are not covered entities under the rule.[73,119]

Although cancer registries are not subject to the Privacy Rule, they must comply with the state cancer registry laws, consisting of statutes and administrative regulations, that authorize their establishment and maintenance and that govern their operations. Almost all of these laws expressly state that information about cancer patients are confidential subject to designated exceptions, and they either explicitly or implicitly restrict its use and limit its disclosure to protect its confidentiality.[7]

In addition, registries may be subject to other state laws that may have some bearing on the confidentiality of registry information. Among these laws are state freedom-of-information acts, or state public records laws, giving the public the right of access to government held information. These laws, which exist in all 50 states, may be superseded by the confidentiality provisions of state cancer registry laws.[120]

12.4.1.2 Confidentiality Protections and Identifiability of Cancer Registry Data

There is an initial question regarding whether the confidentiality of cancer registry information about individual cancer patients should depend on whether the information is individually identifiable. Arguably, the release of nonidentifiable information is not harmful to cancer patients and does not compromise their privacy interests.[39,121] But, insofar as their privacy interests are conceptualized as interests in the ownership and control of the information, the release of nonidentifiable information can be seen as compromising their privacy interests even if its release would not reveal their individual identities.[9]

The prevailing view appears to be that only individually identifiable personal information is deserving of confidentiality protections. This view is reflected in widely accepted national and international standards for the protection of the confidentiality of personal information, including personal health information.[39,58,121,122] This view also is reflected in policies and best practices for the protection of the confidentiality of cancer registry data, including geocoded data, recommended by the North American Association of Central Cancer Registries (NAACCR) and the International Association of Cancer Registries.[4,83,119,123]

At the federal level, a number of laws extend confidentiality protections to identifiable information and do not extend these protections to nonidentifiable information.[54,58] For example, under the HIPAA Privacy Rule, the use and disclosure of protected health information, defined as individually identifiable information, is regulated, and nonidentifiable information is not regulated.[8 at 45 CFR §§ 164.103, 164.514(a)]

The confidentiality provisions of state cancer registry laws vary from state to state. Most registry laws provide, or can be interpreted as providing, that identifiable information is confidential.[7] A few registry laws provide, or can be interpreted as providing, that cancer registry information is confidential whether or not the data is identifiable.[7] Finally, some registry laws do not make clear the scope of their confidentiality protections.[7] See the appendix for a list of state laws.

There are few state court decisions dealing with the confidentiality provisions of state cancer registry laws. In one of the handful of decisions in this area, an Illinois court held that cancer registry data, which a newspaper requested under the Illinois freedom-of-information act, should be released even though a state statute prohibited public release of individually identifiable registry data.[124] The court concluded that the release of the requested registry data by ZIP code, by type of cancer, and by date of diagnosis would not reasonably tend to lead to the identification of specific persons notwithstanding the expert testimony to the contrary.[124]

12.4.1.3 Restrictions on Use of and Access to Registry Data

One approach to protection of the confidentiality of cancer registry data is to impose restrictions on the use of and access to confidential data. Underlying this approach is the principle that confidential data should be used for legitimate purposes and the principle that the persons and the organizational entities, given access to confidential data, should have a demonstrable need to use the data for legitimate purposes.[39,121,122] Legitimate purposes are those directly related to the purposes for which the information was originally collected.[39,122] This means that the use of confidential cancer registry data should be restricted to cancer surveillance and to cancer control and protection activities. This also means that access to data should be restricted to persons and organizational entities with a demonstrable need to use the data for these purposes.

There is great variation in state laws that regulate the use of and access to confidential registry data. The result is a crazy quilt of legal requirements that are not consistent, much less uniform, from state to state.[7] State cancer registry laws that spell out detailed restrictions on the use of and access to confidential data are the exception rather than the rule, and they are all too often ambiguous and outdated.[7] In many states, they do not fully protect the confidential information of cancer patients because they do not adequately restrict the purposes for which this information may be used and who may have access to this information.[7] In other states, they may impede the use of and access to this information for legitimate purposes related to cancer surveillance and cancer prevention and control activities through overly stringent restrictions.[7]

The use of the confidential information of cancer patients for research and the access of research institutions and individual researchers to this information is important for state registry laws to address inasmuch as this information is widely used for epidemiologic, health services, and clinical research.[100] Most state cancer registry laws expressly authorize, or appear to authorize, the external release of confidential information for research.[7] A majority of these laws require some sort of explicit approval prior to the release of confidential information for research.[7] The designated decision makers in this regard variously include an institutional review board (IRB), a research review committee, the state public health agency, and the state public health commissioner or director.[7] Most laws, however, requiring approval lack specificity regarding the criteria to be applied in making approval decisions.[7] Some state laws condition release of confidential information to researchers on confidentiality agreements or assurances of confidentiality protections and prohibit researchers from making secondary disclosures of this information.[7]

A great deal of confusion surrounds the permissibility of using confidential registry data for research because of confusion about the interaction between state registry laws regulating the use of and access to registry data; the HIPAA Privacy Rule regulating the use and disclosure of PHI by covered entities, including health care providers; and the Federal Policy for the Protection of Human Subjects, known as the Common Rule, regulating federally funded human subject research. The HIPAA Privacy Rule, generally prohibiting a covered entity from using or disclosing PHI without individual authorization, contains not only a public health exception but also a research exception to this prohibition. But, the research exception requirements are stricter than the public health exception requirements. The Privacy Rule allows a covered entity to disclose PHI for research purposes without individual authorization if an IRB or a privacy board approves a waiver or alteration of the individual authorization in accordance with certain review criteria.[8 at 45 CFR § 164.512(i) and § 164.514(e)]

The Common Rule applies to organizational entities that conduct research involving human subjects and that receive support from HHS and a number of other federal agencies.[125] The Common Rule defines human subject research as "a systematic investigation, including research development, testing and evaluation, designed to develop or contribute to generalizable knowledge" that involves "a living individual about whom an investigator ... conducting research obtains data through intervention or interaction with the individual, or identifiable private information."[125 at 45 CFR §46.102] Under the Common Rule, organizational entities must establish an IRB, composed of scientists and nonscientists, to review research proposals to determine if research subjects will be appropriately protected.[125 at 45 CFR § 46.103] Among the matters that an IRB must review is whether the privacy of individually identifiable information is properly protected.[125 at 45 CFR § 46.111]

The applicability of the Privacy Rule and the Common Rule to the collection, use, and disclosure of personal health information of cancer patients for cancer surveillance and related epidemiological, health services, and clinical research depends on whether they are characterized and classified as public health practice or research. HHS and other experts have attempted to furnish guidance on how to distinguish between public health practice and research.[70,126,127] For example, the Centers for Disease Control and Prevention (CDC) guidelines state: "If the primary intent is to prevent or control disease or injury and no research is intended at the present time, the project is non-research. If the primary intent changes to generating generalizable knowledge, then the project becomes research."[126] Because an in-depth examination of the distinctions between public health practice and research is beyond the scope of this chapter, suffice it to say that it is not always easy to discern whether an activity belongs in the former or the latter category, and these distinctions sometimes have an "Alice-in-Wonderland" quality.[128]

12.4.1.4   Data Disclosure Limitations

Another approach to protecting the confidentiality of cancer registry data is to limit external disclosure of individually identifiable data to entities and individuals outside the registry. This approach to confidentiality protection is intended to minimize the risk of identification of cancer patients, who are the subjects of registry data files, through data deidentification. Deidentified data are data that have been modified to reduce the potential for identification of individual data subjects.[129] Registries traditionally have released so-called public use files of deidentified data to the public for research purposes and other purposes.[119]

One obvious method of deidentifying registry data is to remove personal identifiers (e.g., name, address, date of birth, social security number, etc.) that may directly identify cancer patients.[119,129] Unfortunately, the removal of personal identifiers is not necessarily sufficient to prevent indirect identification of cancer patients under some circumstances and in some contexts. As the NAACCR Standards for Cancer Registries explain: "Consider a report that indicates that prostate cancer was diagnosed in a 65-year-old African American male in a geographic area whose residents are primarily of Asian ancestry. Even though no confidential information is released, this might allow someone with knowledge of the geographic area to identify the patient."[119 at p. 51]

A related but distinct problem stems from the linkage of registry records with records in other available public and private databases. Record linkage refers to the computer-aided combination of data about specific persons from one source with additional data about the same persons, their associates, and their geographic environment from other sources.[129] Government-conducted and -sponsored record linkage projects have become commonplace in cancer and other health research.[129] The linkage of deidentified data files with other data files may facilitate the reidentification of some data subjects.[119,129]

Various statistical methods have been and are being developed to forestall the indirect, as well as the direct, identification of individual data subjects.[129,130] In connection with these methods, questions exist regarding how to define and measure the identifiability of data files, and in response to these questions NAACCR initiated a Record Uniqueness Program to evaluate registry data files for their potential to identify and reidentify individual cancer patients.[119]

What current disclosure limitation methods can do is to minimize the risk of identification and reidentification of individual data subjects. What these methods cannot do is guarantee that deidentified data will remain so. This is especially true in an era in which the number of electronic databases containing personal information about individuals is constantly growing, and advances in information technology (IT) are constantly making it easier to access and link these databases.[129–131] Moreover, the use of these methods may have a negative impact on the value of data for research and other activities; the more effective these methods are in deidentifying data, the more negative their impact may be on the ability of researchers and others to use the data.[58,130–132]

In formulating and implementing legal standards for the release of registry data, it is necessary to make tradeoffs between apparently conflicting objectives.[58,130–132] One objective is to protect the confidentiality of data and to minimize the risk of direct and indirect identification of individual data subjects after data are released. Other objectives are to maximize data quality and to facilitate data access to accommodate the need for data for legitimate purposes, such as research.

State cancer registry laws by and large furnish little or no direction to registries regarding how to make the necessary tradeoffs between data protection and data quality and access. Many statutes and administrative regulations that prohibit the disclosure of identifiable registry data do not indicate what constitutes identifiable data; conversely, many statutes and administrative regulations that allow the disclosure of nonidentifiable data do not indicate what constitutes nonidentifiable data; some statutes and administrative regulations simply authorize the release of data in a summary, statistical, or aggregate form.[7] The fact that state registry laws fail to provide concrete requirements for deidentification of registry data means that registries have a great deal of latitude regarding their deidentification practices. NAACCR has formulated standards for disclosure of confidential registry data and disseminated information about best practices for deidentification of registry data.[119,123,133] Little information, however, is readily available on policies and practices that registries have voluntarily adopted.

In contrast to state cancer registry laws, the HIPAA Privacy Rule, generally prohibiting covered entities from releasing PHI without individual authorization unless it has been deidentified, sets forth detailed requirements for the deidentification of such information. Although the Privacy Rule does not regulate the use and disclosure of cancer registry data, cancer registry personnel and other persons who work with registry data may look to the rule for guidance regarding appropriate deidentification standards in the absence of state laws that enunciate such standards.

The rule specifies that the requisite deidentification can be accomplished through two different methods. Under the statistical deidentification method, a properly qualified statistician using accepted techniques must conclude that "the risk is very small that the information could be used, alone or in combination with other reasonably available information, by an anticipated recipient to identify an individual who is a subject of the information."[8 at 45 CFR § 164.514(b) (1)] Under the safe harbor method, a covered entity must remove any of 18 individual identifiers from the information, and the covered entity must not have "actual knowledge that the remaining information could be used alone or in combination with other data to identify an individual who is a subject of the information."[8 at 45 CFR § 164.514(b) (2)] The rule also allows covered entities to release limited data sets, with more identifiers than deidentified data sets, for public health, research, or health care operations. But, the rule requires that a covered entity must enter into a data use agreement with the recipient, and that this agreement must enumerate how the data will be used and disclosed and how the data will be protected against impermissible use and disclosure.[8 at 45 CFR § 164.514(e)]

12.4.1.5   Licensing, Secure Sites, and Remote Access

Recognizing that traditional methods of limiting disclosure of confidential data, such as withholding data and altering data, may also limit the utility and value of the data for meaningful and reliable analysis, governmental agencies have begun to explore alternatives to these traditional methods. These alternatives are directed at giving researchers access to confidential data for legitimate research projects for which public use files of deidentified data and limited data sets are not sufficient.[54,134–136]

One alternative is data licensing. Under a data license, or data use agreement, a federal or state agency, holding confidential data, permits qualified and approved research institutions and individual researchers access to its data for a limited time; in exchange, these institutions and individuals agree to abide by the agency's requirements for protection of data confidentiality.[134] The National Cancer Institute and the Centers for Medicare and Medicaid have data use agreements for the Surveillance, Epidemiology, and End Results–Medicare Database (SEER-Medicare).[134]

Other alternatives furnish safe settings and mechanisms for access to confidential data by federal researchers. Several federal data-holding agencies have established secure remote sites and remote access arrangements. With secure remote sites, the data-holding agency retains control of the data, and researchers are afforded access to the data at an agency secure site. At these sites, researchers must comply with the same confidentiality policies and practices as agency personnel.[135] In remote access arrangements, the data-holding agency retains control of the data that researchers access electronically through an intermediary that the agency controls and that is responsible for enforcing compliance with confidentiality requirements.[136]

All of these "access modalities" represent an attempt to maximize data sharing and at the same time to protect the confidentiality of data by allowing data access only under certain conditions or in a controlled environment. The experience of other governmental agencies in planning and implementing these modalities may furnish cancer registries with some models for their use that they can adapt to their own needs. A caveat is that use of these modalities may require changes in statutes and administrative regulations pertaining to the confidentiality of cancer registry information.

12.4.2   CONFIDENTIALITY OF GEOCODED CANCER DATA

The problems associated with protecting the confidentiality of cancer registry data are essentially the same whether or not the data are geocoded. But ensuring the confidentiality of geocoded data does present special challenges.[58] The confidentiality issues related to geocoding that have received the most attention revolve around the risk for direct or indirect identification of individual cancer patients from geocoded data.

When a cancer registry's records are geocoded, a geographic identifier (geocode) is attached to records containing the specific addresses of cancer patients. The resulting geocoded records can be used to create dot or pin maps that show the geographic location of cancer cases. The release of these maps would not seem to constitute a data confidentiality protection problem because they do not directly identify the individuals to whom the mapped cases correspond.[47,48] Yet, specific addresses of individuals may in fact be recoverable from these maps through a process known as reverse geocoding or inverse address matching.[4,47,48,137] The recovered addresses can then be linked to other available databases, such as telephone directories, city directories, and real estate records, to reveal the actual identity of these individuals.[47,48]

Because maps of geocoded cancer registry data and other health data are vulnerable to reverse geocoding, their dissemination poses a threat to data confidentiality. There is a particularly high risk that the public or semipublic dissemination of such maps will compromise data confidentiality. A concomitant of the expansion of the use of GIS technology in public health and health sciences research is a growth in dissemination of maps of geocoded health data through their publication in print, their placement on Internet Web sites, and their presentation in public forums. The number of articles with maps of geocoded patient health data published in medical and other professional journals is illustrative. Publication of such articles is growing at a rate of about 26% each year,[111] and 19 such articles with maps displaying the geographic locations of the cases of more than 19,000 patients were published from 1994 to 2004 in five major medical journals.[138] Some studies have demonstrated that geocoded health data of individuals currently published as low-resolution maps in medical journals, other professional journals, and even newspapers are susceptible to reverse geocoding, and that reverse geocoding can lead to the disclosure of the specific addresses of a substantial proportion of these individuals.[137–139]

Publicly accessible maps of geocoded cancer data from which the specific addresses of cancer patients can be recovered raise the specter that these maps may become a source for data-mining activities for purposes completely unrelated to and inconsistent with public health goals and objectives. Data mining refers to the automated techniques for extracting knowledge from a large volume of data.[140,141] Businesses have engaged in data mining for a number of years, and the federal government is increasingly using data mining.[141] Data-mining efforts are employed to generate highly detailed profiles of individuals based on personal information about them from multiple, formerly separate, public and private sector databases.[33,101] A frequent use of data mining is database marketing — the creation of databases of profiles of individuals that enable businesses to target the marketing of their goods and services effectively and efficiently.[33,101,141,142] It is conceivable that data mining could be used by businesses to target cancer patients for some types of marketing activities. It also is conceivable that data mining could be used by employers to ascertain the health status of cancer patients who are applying for jobs, by insurance companies to ascertain the health status of cancer patients seeking insurance coverage, and by health care facilities to recruit new cancer patients.

Thus far, a major focus of efforts to protect the confidentiality of geocoded data has been the development of methods to deidentify the data before maps derived from the data are released. Conventional methods to deidentify geocoded data entail the aggregation of all address-level records of individuals into a geographic unit with a population large enough to preclude the identification of their exact addresses from a map of geocoded data.[119,143] For example, address-level data might be aggregated into a larger geographic area such as a state, county, census tract, or ZIP code to produce a map showing the distribution of cases on the basis of these units rather than a street basis.

Although the geographic aggregation of geocoded cancer registry data and other health data can protect the confidentiality of the data, the value of the data for some types of analysis may be adversely affected.[143] For example, the aggregation of geo-coded cancer registry data may hinder the ability of researchers to detect local-ized clusters of cancer cases and to investigate the suspected relationship between unusual clusters and environmental exposures.[143–145]

A promising alternative to data aggregation methods are data-masking methods. Such methods are designed to preserve the confidentiality of geocoded cancer data and other health data by minimizing the risk of individual identity disclosure and at the same time to preserve the properties and relationships of the geocoded data that are required for meaningful and reliable data analysis. Masking methods involve the systematic modification of the geographic identifiers assigned to the addresses of individuals in the records geocoded to "mask" the precise location of individual cases. For a description of masking methods and a discussion of their effectiveness see chapters 7 and 8 of this volume.

The utilization of GIS technology in public health and in cancer prevention and control is expanding but is still relatively new. State cancer registry laws usually pre-date the application of GIS technology to cancer registry data. It is not surprising then that state cancer registry laws by and large do not address, much less attempt to resolve, the tension between the objective of protecting the confidentiality of geo-coded data and the objectives of preserving the quality of and facilitating access to geocoded data.[7]

Here again, state cancer registries may turn to the HIPAA Privacy Rule for guid-ance despite the fact that the rule is not applicable to registries. The rule takes an aggregation approach to the deidentification of health information with individual geographic identifiers. It specifies that deidentification requires the removal of "all geographic subdivisions smaller than a State, including street address, city, county, precinct, zip code, and their equivalent geocodes."[8 at 45 CFR 164.514(b)] It however enunci-ates an exception to this requirement if "the geographic unit formed by combining all zip codes with the same three initial digits contains more than 20,000 people," and if "the initial three digits of a zip code for all such geographic units containing 20,000 or fewer people is changed to 000."[8 at 45 CFR 164.514(b)]

In summary, the issues surrounding the protection of the confidentiality of can-cer registry data, including geocoded data, are many and complex. The present state statutes and administrative regulations, which control the way in which registries use and disclose confidential registry data, often fail to address such issues and to demonstrate a real understanding of such issues. These state cancer registry laws, taken as a whole, need to be reexamined and revised. A starting point for such reex-amination and reform are two model acts: the Model State Public Health Privacy Act and the Turning Point Model State Public Health Act, which were the product of the collaboration of public health experts and stakeholders and were developed to stimulate reform of state public health laws.[39,121,146,147]

12.5 REGISTRY DATA AND INFORMATION TECHNOLOGY SECURITY

Even optimal legal requirements for protection of the confidentiality of cancer registry data before, during, and after geocoding may be rendered meaningless if the security of registry data is not adequately safeguarded. Establishment and maintenance of comprehensive, effective information technology (IT) security programs are critically important to protect the confidentiality of registry data. IT security programs consist of administrative, physical, and technical policies, procedures, and practices and mechanisms/methods to protect confidentiality, integrity, reliability, and availability of information and information systems.[8,118] In addition to developing their own IT security programs, cancer registries have a responsibility to take measures to ensure the security of confidential data files that they release to other entities and individuals.

Because of the widespread availability of electronic IT, reports of cancer cases, once submitted in writing to registries, now are usually submitted in an electronic format, and data derived from these reports are routinely stored, retrieved, and transmitted electronically rather than in writing. Arrangements for the security of written records and reports are relatively easy and traditionally took the form of physical safeguards, such as keeping written reports and records in locked rooms and cabinets to which only authorized persons had the key or combination. Arrangements for the security of electronic reports and records is much more complicated and difficult because a large number of data items can be stored on computer files that are easily copied and that can be accessed from and transmitted to computers and computer networks in multiple locations.

Threats to security of registry data may be internal: Personnel who are not authorized to have access to particular confidential data files may nonetheless gain access to such files, and they may make unauthorized disclosures of files. External threats to registry data also abound. One type of external threat comes from outsiders, known as hackers, who may gain entry to confidential data files by attacking and invading Web sites and computer systems through the Internet. Another type of external threat is the potential physical theft of computers, especially laptop computers, and computer equipment with confidential data files.

Breaches of the security of computers and computer systems resulting in unauthorized access to and disclosure of confidential data files have become a major risk in both the public and private sectors. Data security breaches have reportedly compromised millions of identifiable personal records.[148] The number of records compromised has been variously estimated at 90 million during an 18-month period beginning in January 2005, at 100 million in 2005 and 2006, and at 136 million in the 6 years from 2000 to 2006.[148]

In recent years, serious security breaches of federal electronic databases, some of which contain individually identifiable health information, have received a lot of publicity.[149] Federal legislation has been enacted, and executive orders and presidential directives have been issued, aimed at strengthening the security of federal electronic IT systems and public information infrastructures.[150] During 2005, however, a report of the Government Accountability Office (GAO) characterized IT security as a government-wide high-risk area,[151] and a congressional report card gave federal agencies an overall grade of D for IT security.[152]

In 2006, GAO examined the information security practices of the HHS's Centers for Medicare and Medicaid Services (CMS), which oversee the Medicare and Medicaid programs at the federal level. GAO investigators found that CMS had failed to implement effective information security controls over the electronic communication network that it utilizes for transmission of information and data between the CMS central office and CMS-related entities (e.g., CMS regional offices, Medicare intermediaries and carriers, Medicare data centers, state Medicaid offices, private contractors, and subcontractors and health care providers).[153] GAO concluded that the personal health information of Medicare and Medicaid beneficiaries transmitted via the network was at risk for improper disclosure because of numerous security vulnerabilities in the network.[153] Among the vulnerabilities that GAO cited were the failure to use encryption to safeguard sensitive medical data about Medicare and Medicaid beneficiaries, a failure to enforce the use of sufficiently complex password controls for network access, and a failure to audit and monitor the activities of network users for compliance with security policies and procedures.

In 2006, GAO also surveyed private federal contractors responsible for the day-to-day operations of the Medicare program and state Medicaid agencies about security breaches. GAO found security breaches were rampant, with 40% of survey respondents reporting that they had experienced security breaches in the previous 2 years affecting the personal health information of Medicare and Medicaid beneficiaries.[154]

State health agencies also are susceptible to serious security breaches because of a lack of, or deficiencies in, security policies and procedures. A survey of 50 state health agencies published in 1999 found that in a 2-year period one-quarter of these agencies had experienced significant breaches of their electronic information systems, most of which were committed by agency personnel, and that the true number of breaches probably exceeded the number of reported breaches.[155]

Most state statutes and administrative regulations applicable to the operations of population-based central cancer registries are largely silent regarding security policies and procedures for confidential registry data.[7] Only a few have provisions directing cancer registries to adopt measures to safeguard the security of registry data, and these provisions tend to be general.[7]

Even in the absence of state laws and administrative regulations, cancer registries can and should institute IT security programs. Recognizing the importance of preventing breaches of security compromising, or potentially compromising, confidential registry information and data, the NAACCR has sponsored workshops and issued guidance on best practices with respect to security of cancer registry information and data.[123] In developing and implementing IT security programs, cancer registries can draw on NAACCR guidance, other IT security standards, and an extensive body of literature dealing with IT security.[29,118,123,156–160] It is unknown to what extent cancer registries actually have comprehensive and effective IT security programs.

12.6 CONCLUSION

The mandatory reporting of individually identifiable personal health information of cancer patients to state cancer registries and the subsequent use and disclosure of this information raise major privacy, confidentiality, and security concerns.

GIS technology and geocoded data can make a significant contribution to better understanding of geographic patterns of the occurrence of cancer cases and deaths and the relationship between cancer cases and deaths and other variables. But, the use and disclosure of geocoded cancer registry data also present special privacy, confidentiality, and security problems.

Privacy concerns cannot be separated from confidentiality concerns, and privacy and confidentiality concerns cannot be separated from security concerns. They are intrinsically intertwined. Ensuring data confidentiality is necessary to protect data privacy, and safeguarding data security is necessary to protect data confidentiality.

The present legal framework for the reporting of cases to registries and the use and disclosure of registry data consists of numerous federal and state statutes and administrative regulations. These activities, however, are governed primarily by state cancer reporting laws and state cancer registry laws, both statutes and administrative regulations. The privacy, confidentiality, and security provisions of these statutes and regulations, viewed collectively, are deficient in many respects, and they do not give adequate and appropriate direction and guidance to cancer registries. Accordingly, it is important that they undergo review and revision. It is likewise important that the privacy, confidentiality, and security policies and practices voluntarily adopted by cancer registries undergo review and revision.

State public policymakers need to confront and make decisions about many complicated issues that require the accommodation of two sets of conflicting, or at least competing, interests — the interests of cancer patients in the privacy of their personal health information and the interests of the public health function and society in fostering and facilitating cancer surveillance and related cancer prevention and control efforts. It should be recognized, however, that interests of cancer patients and public health and societal interests are not necessarily mutually exclusive and may overlap. Thus, cancer patients may care about reducing the overall cancer burden as well as protecting the privacy of their personal health information. It also behooves public health officials, cancer registry administrators, and users of registry data to protect the privacy of this information to secure the cooperation of cancer patients and their health care providers in conducting cancer surveillance. In short, resolving and reconciling the tensions between interests of cancer patients and public health and societal interests is difficult but not impossible.

REFERENCES

1. National Cancer Institute. *SEER: Surveillance, Epidemiology, and End Results Program*. National Institutes of Health, U.S. Department of Health and Human Services, Bethesda, MD, September 2005.
2. U.S. Department of Health and Human Services, Centers for Disease Control and Prevention. Cancer-NPCR fact sheet. 2006. http://apps.neccd.cdc.gov.
3. U.S. Department of Health and Human Services, Centers for Disease Control and Prevention. Cancer-NPCR cancer surveillance system rationale and approach, n.d.. http://apps.nccd.cdc.gov.
4. Wiggins, I. (Ed.). *Using Geographic Information Systems Technology in the Collection, Analysis and Presentation of Cancer Registry Data: A Handbook of Basic Practices*. North American Association of Cancer Registries, Springfield, IL, 2002.

5. World Health Organization. GIS and public health mapping. (n.d.). http://www.whoint/ health-mapping/gisandphm/en/print.html.

6. Rushton, G. et al. Geocoding in cancer research: a review. *Am. J. Prev. Med.*, 30(2S), S16–S24, 2006.

7. Gittler, J. Compendium of state cancer reporting laws and cancer registry laws. Compendium on file with the National Health Law and Policy Resource Center, College of Law, University of Iowa, Iowa City, 2006.

8. U.S. Department of Health and Human Services. Standards for privacy of individually identifiable health information (Privacy Rule), 45 CFR parts 160 and 164, subparts A and E, 2006.

9. Bezanson, R. Privacy and geocoding: a privacy matrix. Paper on file with the National Health Law and Policy Resource Center, College of Law, University of Iowa, Iowa City, 2004.

10. Cate, F. H. *Privacy in the Information Age*. Brookings Institute, Washington, DC, 1997.

11. Gormley, K. One hundred years of privacy. *Wis. Law Rev.*, 1335–1442, 1992.

12. Solove, D., and Rothenberg, M. *Information Privacy Law*. Aspen, New York, 2003.

13. Solove, D. Conceptualizing privacy. *Calif. Law Rev.*, 90, 1087–1156, 2002.

14. Turkington, R., and Allen, A. *Privacy Law*. 2nd ed. West Group, St. Paul, MN, 2002.

15. Gostin, L.O. Health information privacy. *Cornell Law Rev.* 80, 451–528.

16. U.S. Congress, Office of Technology Assessment. *Protecting Privacy in Computerized Medical Information* (OTA-TCT-576). U.S. Government Printing Office, Washington, DC, 1993.

17. California Healthcare Foundation. *National Consumer Health Privacy Survey 2005*. California Healthcare Foundation, San Francisco, 2005.

18. California Healthcare Foundation. *Medical Privacy and Confidentiality Survey: Summary and Overview*. California Health Care Foundation, San Francisco, January 28, 1999.

19. Electronic Privacy Information Center. *Medical Privacy Public Opinion Polls*. Electronic Privacy Information Center, Washington, DC, n.d.. Also available online at www.epic.org/privacy/medical/polls.html.

20. Gallup Organization. *Public Attitudes toward Medical Privacy*. Institute for Health Freedom, Washington, DC, 2000. Also available online at http://forhealthfreedom.org/ Gallup survey/IHf-Gallup.html.

21. Health Privacy Project. *Health Privacy Polling Data*. Health Privacy Project, Washington, DC, n.d.

22. National Committee on Vital and Health Statistics. *Privacy and Confidentiality in the Nationwide Health Information Network*. National Committee on Vital and Health Statistics, Washington, DC, 2006. Also available online at www.ncvhs.hhs.gov/060622lt.html.

23. Westin, A. F. *How the Public Views Health Privacy: Survey Results from 1978 to 2005*. Program on Information Technology, Health Records and Privacy, Center for Social and Legal Research, Hackensack, NJ, February 23, 2005.

24. National Research Council. *For the Record: Protecting Electronic Health Information*. National Academy Press, Washington, DC, 1997.

25. Reiser, S. J., Dyck, A. J., and Curran, W. J. *Ethics in Medicine: Historical Perspectives and Contemporary Concerns*. MIT Press, Cambridge, MA, 1977, chap. 1.

26. American Medical Association, Council on Ethical and Judicial Affairs. *Code of Medical Ethics, Current Opinions with Annotations*. 2004–2005 ed. AMA Press, Chicago, 2004, chap. 5.

27. American Nurses Association. *Code of Ethics for Nurses with Interpretative Statements*. Nursebooks.org, Silver Springs, MD, 2001.

28. California Healthcare Foundation and Consumers Union. *Promoting Health, Protecting Privacy: A Primer*. California Health Care Foundation, San Francisco, 1999.

29. U.S. Department of Health and Human Services. Standards for privacy of individually identifiable health information; Final Rule, Background. 65 Federal Register (Fed. Reg.) 82463–82474, December 28, 2000.

30. Agre, P. E. and Rothenberg, M. (Eds.). *Technology and Privacy: The New Landscape*. MIT Press, Cambridge, MA, 1997.

31. Flaherty, D. H. *Protecting Privacy in Surveillance Societies*. University of North Carolina Press, Chapel Hill, 1989.

32. Garfinkel, S. *Database Nation: The Death of Privacy in the 21st Century*. O'Reilly Media, North Sebastopol, CA, 2000.

33. Kang, J. Information privacy in cyberspace transactions. *Stanford Law Rev.,* 50, 1193–1294, 1998.

34. Karas, S. Privacy, identity, databases. *Am. Univ. Law Rev.,* 52, 393, 2002.

35. Katsh, M. E. *Law in a Digital World*. Oxford University Press, New York, 1995.

36. Miller, A. *The Assault on Privacy*. University of Michigan Press, Ann Arbor, 1971.

37. O'Harrow, R., Jr. *No Place to Hide*. Free Press, New York, 2005.

38. Westin, A. F. *Privacy and Freedom*. Atheneum, New York, 1967.

39. Gostin, L., Hodge, J. G., and Valdiserri, R. O. Informational privacy and the public's health: the model state public health privacy act. *Am. J. Public Health,* 91, 1388–1392, 2001.

40. Gostin, L. et al. The public health information infrastructure: a national review of the law on health information policy. *JAMA,* 275, 1921–1927, 1996.

41. Gostin, L. and Hodge, J. G. Personal privacy and common goods: a framework for balancing under the national health information privacy rule. *Minn. Law Rev.,* 86, 1439–1480, 2002.

42. Health Privacy Project. *Health Information Technology — Consumer Principles*. Health Privacy Project, Washington, DC, March 2006. Also available online at http://www.healthprivacy.org.

43. Institute of Medicine, Committee on Regional Health Networks. *Health Data in the Information Age: Use, Disclosure, and Privacy*, Donaldson, M. S., and Lohr, K. N., Eds. National Academy Press, Washington, DC, 1994.

44. Rybowski, L. *Protecting the Confidentiality of Health Information*. National Health Policy Forum, George Washington University, Washington, DC, July 1998.

45. U.S. General Accounting Office. *Medical Records Privacy, Access Needed for Health Research, But Oversight of Privacy Is Limited* (GAO/HEHS-99-55). U.S. General Accounting Office, Washington, DC, February 1999.

46. Anselin, L. How not to lie with spatial statistics. *Am. J. Prev. Med.,* 30(2S), S3–S6, 2006.

47. Armstrong, M. P. Geographic information technologies and their potentially erosive effects on personal privacy. *Stud. Soc. Sci.,* 27, 19–28, 2002.

48. Armstrong, M. P., and Ruggles, A. L. Geographic information technologies and personal privacy. *Cartographica,* 40(4), 63–73, 2005.

49. Curry, M. R. In plain and open view: geographic information systems and the problem of privacy. In *Proceedings of the Conference on Law and Information Policy for Spatial Databases*, National Center for Geographic Information and Analysis, Orono, ME, pp. 212–218, 1995.

50. Curry, M. R. Rethinking privacy in a geocoded world. In *Geographical Information Systems: Principles, Techniques, Applications and Management*. Longley, P. A., et al., Eds. Wiley, New York, 1999, Vol. 2, chap. 55.

51. Curry, M. R. The digital individual and the private realm. *Ann. Assoc. Am. Geogr.,* 87, 681–699, 1997.

52. Dobson, J. Is GIS a privacy threat? *GeoWorld,* 11(7), 34–35, 1998.

53. Dobson, J. and Fisher, P. Geoslavery, *IEEE Technol. Soc.,* Spring, 47–52, 2003.

54. Golden, M. L., Downs, R. R., and Davis-Packard, K. *Confidentiality Issues and Policies Related to the Utilization and Dissemination of Geospatial Data for Public Health Applications*. Socioeconomic Data and Applications Center, Center for International Earth Science Information Network, Columbia University, Palisades, 2005.
55. Goss, J. We know who you are and we know where you live: the instrumental rationality of geodemographic systems. *Econ. Geogr.*, 71, 171–198, 1995.
56. Matthews, S. A. *GIS and Privacy* (GIS Resource Document 03-51). Pennsylvania State University, State College, PA, 2003.
57. Monmonier, M. *Spying with Maps: Surveillance Technologies and the Future of Privacy*. University of Chicago Press, Chicago, 2002.
58. National Research Council. *Putting People on the Map: Protecting Confidentiality with Linked Social Spatial Data*. Guttman, M. P., and Stern, P. C., Eds. National Academy Press, Washington, D.C. 2007.
59. Onsrud, H., Johnson, J. P., and Lopez, X. Protecting personal privacy in using geographic information systems. *Photogram. Eng. Remote Sens.*, 60, 1083–1095, 1994.
60. Onsrud, H. and Reis, R. Law and information policy for spatial databases: a research agenda. *Jurimetr. J.*, 35, 377, 1995.
61. VanWey, L. K. et al. Confidentiality and spatially explicit data: concerns and challenges. *Proc. Natl. Acad. Sci. U. S. A.*, 102, 15337–15342, 2005.
62. Waters, N. GIS and the bitter fruit: privacy issues in the age of the Internet. *GeoWorld* [series on the Internet], August 6, 2005. www.geoplace.com/gw/2000/0500/0500edg.asp.
63. Goldman, J. Protecting privacy to improve health care. *Health Aff.,* 17(6), 47–60, 1998.
64. Westin, A. F. Public attitudes towards electronic records. *Privacy and American Business, Electronic Newsletter,* 1–5, February 2005.
65. Grad, F. P. *The Public Health Law Manual*, 3rd ed. American Public Health Association, Washington, DC, 2005, chaps. 4 and 5.
66. Pritts, J. L Altered states: state health privacy laws and the impact of the federal privacy rule. *Yale J. Health Pol'y Law & Ethics*, 2, 327–364, 2002.
67. Pritts, J. *The State of Health Privacy: An Uneven Terrain, a Comprehensive Survey of State Health Privacy Statutes*. Health Privacy Project, Institute for Health Care Research and Policy, Georgetown University, Washington, DC, 1999.
68. Pritts, J. L., et al. *The State of Health Privacy, a Survey of State Health Privacy Statutes,* 2nd ed. Institute for Health Care, Research and Policy, Georgetown University, Washington, DC, 2002.
69. *Health Insurance Portability and Accountability Act of 1996 (HIPAA)*, Pub. L. No. 104-191 §§ 261–264 (1996), most sections codified at 42 U.S.C. §§ 1320d–1320d-8 (2006).
70. U.S. Department of Health and Human Services, National Institute of Health. *Protecting Personal Health Information in Research: Understanding the HIPAA Privacy Rule*, 2003.
71. Deapen, D. Cancer surveillance and information: balancing public health with privacy and confidentiality concerns (United States). *Cancer Causes Control,* 17, 633–637, 2006.
72. Centers for Disease Control and Prevention. HIPAA privacy rule and public health, guidance from CDC and the U.S. Department of Health and Human Services, *MMWR Morb. Mortal. Wkly. Rep.,* 52(suppl) 17, 19–20, 2003.
73. North American Association of Central Cancer Registries. *Frequently Asked Questions and Answers about Cancer Reporting and the HIPAA Privacy Rule*. North American Association of Central Cancer Registries, Springfield, IL, March 31, 2003.
74. *Cancer Registries Amendment Act*, P. L. No. 102-515, 106 Stat. 3372, codified at 42 U.S.C. §§ 280e, 280e-1 to 280e-4 (2003).
75. Bayer, R. and Fairchild, A. L. Surveillance and privacy. *Science*, 290, 1898–1899, 2000.

76. Gittler, J. The resurgence of tuberculosis and public health control measures: challenges for public policy makers. *J. Health Politics Policy Law,* 19, 107–147, 1994.
77. Iverson, A. et al. Consent, confidentiality and the Data Protection Act. *BMJ,* 332, 165–169, 2006.
78. Verity, C. and Nicholl, A. Consent, confidentiality, and the threat to public health surveillance. *BMJ,* 324, 1210–1213, 2002.
79. Brown, P. Cancer registries fear imminent collapse. *BMJ,* 321, 849, 2000.
80. Chantler, C. Informed consent for cancer registration. *Lancet Oncol.,* 2, 8, 2001.
81. Illman, J. Cancer registries: should informed consent be required? *J. Natl. Cancer Inst.,* 94, 1269–1270, 2002.
82. United Kingdom Association of Cancer Registries. Statement by the U.K. Association of Cancer Registries (UKACR) on the General Medical Council (GMC) guidance on confidentiality. *BMJ.,* 321, 854, 2000.
83. International Association of Cancer Registries (IACR). *Guidelines on Confidentiality for Population-Based Cancer Registration.* IACR, Lyon, France, 2004.
84. Barrett, G. et al. National survey of British public views on use of identifiable medical data by the National Cancer Registry. *BMJ,* 332, 1068–1072, 2006.
85. Clark, A. M. and Findley, I. A. Attaining adequate consent for the use of electronic patient records: an opt-out strategy to reconcile individuals' rights and public benefit. *Public Health,* 119, 1003–1010, 2005.
86. Jacobsen, S. J. et al. Potential effect of authorization bias on medical record research. *Mayo Clin. Proc.,* 74, 330–338, 1999.
87. Armstrong, B. A. et al. Potential impact of the HIPAA Privacy Rule on data collection in a registry of patients with acute coronary syndrome. *Arch. Intern. Med.,* 165, 1125–1129, 2005.
88. Dudeck, J. Informed consent for cancer registration. *Lancet Oncol.,* 2, 8–9, 2000.
89. Gorby, N. S., Wolf, M. S., and Bennett, C. L. Introducing HIPAA: triple the cost and triple the time for patient recruitment to the SELECT study. *2004 ASCO Annu. Meet. Proc. J. Clin. Oncol.,* 22(14S), 6009, 2004.
90. Nosowsky, R. and Giordano, T. J. The Health Insurance Portability and Accountability Act of 1996 (HIPPA) Privacy Rule: implications for clinical research. *Annu. Rev. Med.,* 57, 575–590, 2006.
91. Tu, J. V. et al. Impracticability of informed consent in the registry of the Canadian stroke network. *N. Engl. J. Med.,* 350, 1414–1421, 2004.
92. Hewison, J. and Haines, A. Confidentiality and consent in medical research: overcoming barriers to recruitment in health research. *BMJ.,* 333, 300–302, 2006.
93. Junhans, C. et al. Recruiting patients to medical research; double-blind randomized trial of "opt-in" versus "opt-out" strategies. *BMJ.,* 331, 940–942, 2005.
94. Trevena, L., Irwig, L., and Barratt, A. Impact of privacy legislation on the number and characteristics of people who are recruited for research: a randomized, controlled trial. *J. Med. Ethics,* 32, 473–477, 2006.
95. Menck, H. R., and Phillips, J. L. Central cancer registries. In *Cancer Registry Management: Principles and Practices,* Hutchinson, C. L. et al., Eds. Kendall/Hunt, Dubuque, IA, 2004, chap. 34.
96. Gerber, E. The privacy context of survey response: an ethnographic account. In *Confidentiality, Disclosure and Data Access, Theory and Practical Applications for Statistical Agencies,* Doyle, P. et al., Eds. Elsevier Science, Amsterdam, 2001, chap. 15.
97. Thacker, S. B. Historical development. In *Principles and Practice of Public Health Surveillance,* 2nd ed., Teutsch, S. M. and Churchill, R. E., Eds. Oxford University Press, New York, 2000.
98. Heymann, D. L. (Ed.). *Control of Communicable Diseases Manual,* 18th ed. American Public Health Association Press, Washington, DC, 2005.

99. U.S. Department of Health and Human Services, Centers for Disease Control and Prevention (CDC). *Preventing and Controlling Cancer: The Nation's Leading Cause of Death, at a Glance 2006*. CDC, Atlanta, 2006.

100. U.S. Department of Health and Human Services. *Healthy People 2010, Understanding and Improving Health*, 2nd ed. U.S. Government Printing Office, Washington, DC, 2000, Vol. 1, chap. 3.

101. U.S. Department of Commerce, National Telecommunications and Information Administration. *Privacy and the NII: Safeguarding Telecommunications-Related Personal Information*. U.S. Department of Commerce, Washington, DC, 1995.

102. Cromley, E. K. GIS and disease. *Annu. Rev. Public Health*, 24, 7–24, 2003.

103. Cromley, E. K. and McLafferty, S. L. *GIS and Public Health*. Guilford Press, New York, 2002.

104. McLafferty, S. L. GIS and health care. *Annu. Rev. Public Health*, 24, 25–42, 2003.

105. Mullner, R. M. et al. Geographic information systems in public health and medicine. *J. Med. Syst.*, 28, 215–221, 2004.

106. Ricketts, T. C. Geographic information systems and public health. *Annu. Rev. Public Health*, 24, 1–6, 2003.

107. Rushton, G. Public health, GIS, and spatial analytic tools. *Annu. Rev. Public Health*, 24, 43–56, 2003.

108. Curtis, A. and Leiter, M. *Geographic Information Systems and Public Health*. IRM Press, Hershey, PA, 2006.

109. National Cancer Institute. Introduction to GIS at NCI. http://www.gis.cancer.gov/nca/.

110. Pickle, L. W. et al. The crossroads of GIS and health information: workshop on developing a research agenda to improve cancer control. *Int. J. Health Geogr.*, 5, 51, 2006.

111. Pickle, L. W., Waller, L. A., and Lawson, A. B. Current practices in cancer spatial data analysis: a call for guidance. *Int. J. Health Geogr.*, 4, 3, 2005.

112. Klasen, A. C. and Platz, E. A. What can geography tell us about prostate cancer? *Am. J. Prev. Med.*, 30(2S), S7–S15, 2006.

113. Last, J. M. (Ed.). *A Dictionary of Epidemiology*, 4th ed. Oxford University Press, New York, 2000.

114. Johnson, S. *The Ghost Map, the Story of London's Most Terrifying Epidemic — and How It Changed Science, Cities and the Modern World*. Riverhead Books, Penguin Groups, New York, 2006.

115. Clarke, C. C., McLafferty, S. L., and Tempalski, B. J. On epidemiology and geographic information systems: a review and discussion on future directions. *Emerg. Infect. Dis.*, 2, 85–92, 1996.

116. Watkins, S. Legal and ethical aspects of cancer data. In *Cancer Registry Management: Principles and Practice*, Hutchinson, C. L. et al., Eds. Kendall/Hunt, Dubuque, IA, 2004, chap. 5.

117. U.S. Information Infrastructure Task Force, Privacy Working Group. *Privacy and the National Information Infrastructure: Principles for Providing and Using Personal Information*. Executive Office of the President, Office of Management and Budget, Washington, DC, 1995.

118. U.S. Information Infrastructure Task Force, Security Issues Forum. *NII Security: The Federal Role at 2*. Executive Office of the President, Office of Management and Budget, Washington, DC, 1995.

119. North American Association of Central Cancer Registries. *Standards for Cancer Registries Volume 3: Standards for Completeness, Quality, Analysis, and Management of Data*, Havener L., Ed. North American Association of Central Cancer Registries, Springfield, IL, October 2004.

120. The Freedom of Information Center. State FOI laws. http://foi.missouri.edu/index.html.

121. Model State Public Health Privacy Project. *Model State Public Health Privacy Act — with Comments* [final draft]. Center for Law and the Public's Health at Georgetown and Johns Hopkins Universities, Baltimore, MD, 1999.

122. Organization for Economic Co-operation and Development (OECD). Council recommendation concerning guidelines governing the protection of privacy and transborder flows of personal data, 20 I.L.M. 422 (1981), OECD Doc. C (80) 58 (Final), October 1, 1980.

123. North American Association of Central Cancer Registries. *NAACCR Workshop Report: Data Security and Confidentiality.* North American Association of Central Cancer Registries, Springfield, IL, 2002.

124. *The Southern Illinoisan v. Illinois Department of Public Health*, 812 N.E.2d 27 (Ill. App. Ct. 2004).

125. U.S. Department of Health and Human Services. 45CFR, part 46, subpart A (§§ 46.101 to 46.409), 2007.

126. Centers for Disease Control and Prevention. Guidelines for defining public health research and public health non-research. http://www.cdc.gov/od/ads/opspoll1.htm.

127. Hodge, J. G. and Gostin, L. O. *Public Health Practice versus Research, a Report for Public Health Practitioners Including Cases and Guidance for Making Distinctions.* Johns Hopkins Bloomberg School of Public Health, Center for Law and the Public's Health, Baltimore, MD, 2004.

128. Fairchild, A. L. Dealing with Humpty Dumpty: research, practice and the ethics of public health research. *J. Law Med. Ethics*, 331, 615–623, 2003.

129. U.S. General Accounting Office (GAO). *Record Linkage and Privacy, Issues in Creating New Federal Research and Statistical Information* (GAO-01-126SP). GAO, Washington, DC, April 2001.

130. Doyle, P. et al. (Eds.). *Confidentiality, Disclosure, and Data Access, Theory and Practical Applications for Statistical Agencies.* Elsevier Science, Amsterdam, 2001.

131. National Committee on Vital and Health Statistics, Subcommittee on Privacy and Confidentiality. Roundtable discussion: identifiability of data. January 28, 1998. http://ncvhs.hhs.gov/980128tr.htm.

132. Lane, J. *Key Issues in Confidentiality Research: Results of an NSF Workshop.* Urban Institute, Washington, DC, n.d.

133. North American Association of Cancer Registries. *NACCR Workshop Report: North of the Border Workshop I, Surveillance Data Access and Confidentiality Protection in Canadian Cancer Registries.* North American Association of Cancer Registries, Springfield, IL, 2002.

134. Seastrom, M. M. Licensing. In *Confidentiality, Disclosure, and Data Access: Theory and Practical Applications for Statistical Agencies.* Doyle, P. et al., Eds. Elsevier, Amsterdam, 2001, chap. 11.

135. Dunne, T. Issues in the establishment and management of secure sites. In *Confidentiality, Disclosure, and Data Access: Theory and Practical Applications.* Elsevier, Amsterdam, 2001, chap. 12.

136. Blakemore, M. The potential and perils of remote access. In *Confidentiality, Disclosure, and Data Access: Theory and Practical Applications.* Elsevier, Amsterdam, 2001, chap. 13.

137. Curtis, A. J., Mills, J. W., and Leitner, M. Spatial confidentiality and GIS: re-engineering mortality locations from published maps about Hurricane Katrina. *Int. J. Health Geogr.*, 5, 44, 2006.

138. Brownstein, J. S. et al. An unsupervised classification method for inferring original cases locations from low-resolution disease maps. *Int. J. Health Geogr.*, 5, 56, 2006.

139. Brownstein, J. S. Cassa, C. A., and Mandl, K. D. No place to hide — reverse identification of patients from published maps. *N. Engl. J. Med.*, 355, 1741–1742, 2007.

140. Tavani, H. T. Informational privacy, data mining and the Internet. *Ethics Inf. Technol.,* 1, 137–145, 1999.

141. U.S. Government Accountability Office (GAO). *Data Mining: Agencies Have Taken Key Steps to Protect Privacy in Selected Efforts, But Significant Compliance Issues Remain* (GAO-05-866). GAO, Washington, DC, 2005.

142. Linert, K. A. Database marketing and personal privacy in the information age. *Suffolk Transnatl. Law Rev.,* 18, 687–710, 1995.

143. Armstrong, M. P., Rushton, G., and Zimmerman, D. L. Geographically masking health data to preserve confidentiality. *Stat. Med.,* 18, 497–523, 1999.

144. Cassa, C. A. et al. A context sensitive approach to anonymizing spatial surveillance data: impact on outbreak detection. *J. Am. Med. Inform. Assoc.,* 13, 160–165, 2006.

145. Olson, K. L., Grannis, S. J., and Mandl, K. D. Privacy protection versus cluster detection in spatial epidemiology. *Am. J. Public Health,* 96, 2002–2008, 2006.

146. Turning Point Public Health Statute Modernization National Collaborative. *Turning Point Model Public Health Act.* Center for Law and the Public's Health, Georgetown and Johns Hopkins University, Baltimore, MD, 2003.

147. Hodge, J. G. et al. Transforming public health law: the turning point model state public health act. *J. Law Med. Ethics,* 34, 77–84, 2006.

148. Zeller, T., Jr. An ominous milestone: 100 million data leaks. *New York Times,* December 18, 2006, p. C3.

149. Goldfarb, Z. A. To agency insiders, cyber thefts and slow response are no surprise. *Washington Post,* July 18, 2006, p. A17.

150. Moteff, J. *Computer Security: A Summary of Selected Federal Laws, Executive Orders, and Presidential Directives.* Congressional Research Service, Library of Congress, Washington, DC, April 16, 2004.

151. U.S. Government Accountability Office (GAO). *High-Risk Series, an Update* (GAO-05-207), GAO, Washington, DC, January 2005.

152. Davis, T. *News Release: Davis Statement on 2004 Federal Computer Security Report Card Grades.* U.S. House of Representatives, Committee on Government Reform, Washington, DC, February 16, 2005.

153. U.S. Government Accountability Office (GAO). *Information Security, the Centers for Medicare and Medicaid Services Needs to Improve Controls over Key Communication Network* (GAO-06-750). GAO, Washington, DC, August 2006.

154. U.S. Government Accountability Office (GAO). *Domestic and Offshore Outsourcing of Personal Information in Medicare, Medicaid and Tricare* (GAO-06-676). GAO, Washington, DC, 2006.

155. O'Brien, D. G. and Yasnoff, W. A. Privacy, confidentiality and security in information systems of state health agencies. *Am. J. Prev. Med.,* 16, 351–358, 1995.

156. Leestama, R. Implementing technological safeguards to ensure patient privacy. *Caring,* 25(2), 16–18, 2003.

157. Panko, R. *Corporate Computer and Network Security.* Prentice Hall, Upper Saddle River, NJ, 2004.

158. Faris, T. H. *Health Information and Security in Cancer Registry Management: Principles and Practices,* Hutchinson, C. L., et al., Eds. Kendall/Hunt, Dubuque, IA, 2004, chap. 4.

159. Ilioudis, C. and Panaglos, G. A framework for an institutional high level security policy for the processing of medical data and their transmission through the Internet. *J. Med. Internet Res.,* 3(2), e14, 2001.

160. U.S. Department of Health and Human Services. Security standards for the protection of electronic protected health information. 45 CFR parts 160, 162 and 164, subpart C. (§§ 164.302, -304, -306, -308, -310, -312, -314, -316, -318), 2006.

13 Conclusions

Gerard Rushton, Marc P. Armstrong, Josephine Gittler, Barry R. Greene, Claire E. Pavlik, Michele M. West, and Dale L. Zimmerman

Coding the locations of cancer incidences, facilities, and services is now seen as the basis for measuring important aspects of the cancer burden. Standards for assigning these geocodes have not yet been developed, and as this book has shown, there are reasons why this is the case. First among these reasons is the fact that there is no agreement on all of the purposes of geographical analyses of cancer, and if there is agreement regarding purpose, then there is no agreement on the methods of meeting the purpose. However, some conclusions can be reached about good ways to proceed. It is clear that different geocodes are good for serving different purposes, which quickly leads to a conclusion that the question of the best geocode is not an appropriate question. One geocode in particular, the latitude and longitude coordinates of the residence of an individual with cancer, can be the basis of many other geocodes. One way forward is to make the location coordinates of the individual the basic geocode from which other geocodes are developed. Each geocode is valuable to the degree that its use adds value to some purpose. One current problem is that currently available geocodes for cancer become constraints for reaching a given purpose. Current uses of cancer geocodes are thus not a good measure of their future value.

A second reason is that current geocodes are often not complete, and there is concern about errors made in assigning correct geocodes to an incident. A strong and valuable current theme is concern about errors of both omission and commission. The result is many recent studies that have documented these errors in specific situations. More important than any particulars is the fact that a large percentage of these errors can be traced back to errors that were made in recording the address in the first place. There is an emerging consensus that there is need for a better process for initial recording of addresses of cancer incidences. It is now technically possible to verify at the time of original recording whether a given address is valid. These methods are widely used in mass marketing. They could be routinely used in the cancer registration process as they are beginning to be used in some states to register births and deaths.

Each use of a geocode should be examined with respect to the value it adds to the purpose it is addressing. Could some other geocode better meet the purpose — recognizing that location is often used as the attribute to link data together? When location is an attribute for linking datasets, selecting the best geocode becomes more complex because the subordinate purpose — data linkage — is done to meet a more utilitarian purpose related to a substantive cancer purpose. It will not always be clear to the cancer specialist how one geocode may perform better than another when the purpose is to make linkages between datasets that are essentially geospatial linkages.

As the chapter on privacy makes clear, releasing cancer data to the public in the United States occurs within a complex system of state laws, and there undoubtedly will be situations when concerns for privacy will prevent release of cancer data to anyone outside the cancer registration process. This may have a particular impact on the ability to map cancer rates at finer levels of geographic resolution. One possible solution to this problem is to embed the data-processing algorithms within the cancer register computing system and to produce the results of the analysis process in a form that protects the privacy of individuals. These may well be more useful than results of analyses performed on deidentified datasets.

There are consequences of not moving forward in addressing the problems of improving geocodes for cancer data. The most serious include the following: The effectiveness of a great deal of current research on many questions about the cancer burden is substantially reduced because it is using currently available geocodes rather than other geocodes that could have been possible but were not available to the researchers. One current research theme is to identify gradients of change in cancer rates by searching for breaks in rates between county boundaries. But, why should one search the areas between counties? Is it because current cancer data are geocoded so that such searches are possible? There are few studies of the accessibility of cancer patients to treatment facilities. This is surely not because such studies are not needed but because appropriately geocoded data are not available, and the cancer community is not familiar with the spatial analysis methods that can be used in such studies.

If these problems are to be addressed in the future and solved, a better-educated public health workforce will be needed. What this workforce will need to know and how institutions will need to change to deliver this knowledge to the appropriate groups are important questions.

Arizona
    Statutes (Arizona Revised Statutes Annotated [West])
        Ariz. Rev. Stat. Ann. § 36-132 (West 2003 and Supp. 2005)
        Ariz. Rev. Stat. Ann. §§ 36-133 (West 2003)
    Administrative Codes (Arizona Administrative Code)
        Ariz. Admin. Code §§ R9-4-101 to -103, R9-4-201 to -205, R9-4-301 to -303, R9-4-401 to -405 (Supp. 05-2)
Arkansas
    Statutes (West's Arkansas Code Annotated)
        Ark. Code Ann. § 20-15-201 to -204, -206 to -211 (West 2005)
    Administrative Codes (Code of Arkansas Rules [Weil])
        007 14 Ark. Code R. § 007 (Weil 2006)
California
    Statutes (West's Annotated California Codes)
        Cal. Health and Safety Code § 103875, § 103885 (West 2006)
    Administrative Codes (Barclays Official California Code of Regulations)
        Cal. Code Regs. tit. 17, § 2593 (2006)
Colorado
    Statutes (West's Colorado Revised Statutes Annotated)
        Colo. Rev. Stat. Ann. §§ 25-1-122, 25-1.5-102 (West 2006)
    Administrative Codes (Code of Colorado Regulations [Weil])
        6 Colo. Code Regs. § 1009-6 (Weil 2006)
Connecticut
    Statutes (Connecticut General Statutes Annotated [West])
        Conn. Gen. Stat. Ann. § 19a-73 (West 2003)
        Conn. Gen. Stat. Ann. § 19a-215 (West 2003 and Supp. 2006)
    Administrative Codes (Regulations of Connecticut State Agencies)
        Conn. Agencies Regs. § 19a-215-1 to -4 (1992)
Delaware
    Statutes (West's Delaware Code Annotated)
        Del. Code Ann. tit. 16, §§ 3201 to 3203 (West 2003)
    Administrative Codes (Code of Delaware Regulations [Weil])
        16 000 Del. Code Regs. 004 (Weil 2006)

228

Arizona
   Statutes (Arizona Revised Statutes Annotated)
       Ariz. Rev. Stat. Ann. §36-133 (2003)
   Administrative Code (Arizona Administrative Code)
       Ariz. Admin. Code §§ 9-4-104, -401 to -403 (Supp. 2003)

Arkansas
   Statutes (Arkansas Code of 1987 Annotated)
       Ark. Code Ann. §§ 20-15-201 to -205 (2005)
   Administrative Code (Code of Arkansas Rules [Weil])
       007-00-009 Ark. Code. R. §§ 1-8 (Weil 2000)

California
   Statutes (West's Annotated California Codes)
       Cal. Health and Safety Code §§ 103875–103885 (West 2006)
       Cal. Health and Safety Code §§ 104175–104189 (West 2006)
   Administrative Codes (Barclay's California Code of Regulations)
       Cal. Code Regs. tit. 17, § 2593 (Barclays 2006)

Colorado
   Statutes (Colorado Revised Statutes [LexisNexis])
       Colo. Rev. Stat. § 25-1.5 to -.101 (2005)
       Colo. Rev. Stat. § 25-1-122 (2005)
       Colo. Rev. Stat. § 25-1-1202 (2005)
   Administrative Code (Code of Colorado Regulations [Weil])
       6 Colo. Code Regs. § 1009-3 (1995)

Connecticut
   Statutes (General Statutes of Connecticut)
       Conn. Gen. Stat. § 19a-72, -74 (2005)
   Administrative Codes (Regulations of Connecticut State Agencies)
       Conn. Agencies Regs. § 19a-2a-10 (2000)
       Conn. Agencies Regs. § 19a-73-1 to -7 (2000)

Delaware
   Statutes (Delaware Code Annotated [LexisNexis])
       Del. Code Ann. tit. 16 § 3201-08 (2003)
   Administrative Codes (Code of Delaware Regulations [Weil])
       16-4000-4201 Del. Code Regs. § 1–9 (Weil 2005)

District of Columbia
   Statutes (District of Columbia Code Annotated)
       D.C. Code Ann. § 7-301 to -304 (2001)
   Administrative Codes (D.C. Municipal Regulations)
       D.C. Code Mun. Regs. tit. 22 § 125.1 to -.5 (Weil 2000)
       D.C. Code Mun. Regs. tit. 22 § 215.1 to -.4 (Weil 2000)
       D.C. Code Mun. Regs. tit. 22 § 216.1 to -.2 (Weil 2000)
       D.C. Code Mun. Regs. tit. 22 § 217.1 to -.2 (Weil 2000)
       D.C. Code Mun. Regs. tit. 22 § 218.1 to -.2 (Weil 2000)
       D.C. Code Mun. Regs. tit. 22 § 299.1 (Weil 2000)

Florida
    Statutes (Florida Statutes)
        Fla. Stat. § 385.202 (2005)
        Fla. Stat. § 381.0031 (2005)
        Fla. Stat. § 1004.435 (2005)
    Administrative Codes (Florida Administrative Code Annotated)
        Fla. Admin. Code Ann. r. 64D-3.002 to -.006 (2003)

Georgia
    Statutes (Official Code of Georgia Annotated [LexisNexis])
        Ga. Code Ann. §§ 13-12-1, -2 (2006)
        Ga. Code Ann. § 13-15-5 (2006)
    Administrative Codes (Official Compilation Rules and Regulations of the
    State of Georgia)
        Ga. Comp. R. and Regs. 290-5-10.04 (1996)
        Ga. Comp. R. and Regs. 290-5-3-.02, -.03 (2003)

Hawaii
    Statutes (Hawaii Revised Statutes)
        Haw. Rev. Stat. § 321-43 (1993)
        Haw. Rev. Stat. §§ 324-21 to -32 (1997 and Supp. 2005)
    Administrative Codes (Weil's Code of Hawaii Rules)
        None found

Idaho
    Idaho Code Annotated (LexisNexis)
        Idaho Code Ann. § 57-1701 to -1707 (2002)
    Administrative Code (Idaho Administrative Code)
        Idaho Admin. Code r. 16.02.10.010, .020 (2006)
        Idaho Admin. Code r. 16.05.01.001 to -.191 (2006)

Illinois
    Statutes (Illinois Compiled Statutes)
        20 Ill. Comp. Stat. 2310/2310-365 (2004)
        40 Ill. Comp. Stat. 525/1-/14 (2004)
    Administrative Code (Illinois Administrative Code)
        None found

Indiana
    Statutes (Indiana Code)
        Ind. Code § 16-38-2-1 to -9 (1997 and Supp. 2006)
    Administrative Codes (Indiana Administrative Code)
        410 Ind. Admin. Code 21-1-1 to -6 (2001)

Iowa
    Statutes (Code of Iowa)
        Iowa Code § 135.40 to -.41 (2005)
        Iowa Code § 139A.3 (2005)
        Iowa Code § 263.17 (2005)
    Administrative Codes (Iowa Administrative Code)
        Iowa Admin. Code r. 441-9.11 to -.12 (2004)

Iowa Admin. Code r. 641-203.3 (2004)
Iowa Admin. Code r. 641-1.1 to -.6 (2001)

Kansas
    Statutes (Kansas Statutes Annotated)
        Kan. Stat. Ann. §§ 65-1,168 to -1,174 (LexisNexis 2006)
    Administrative Codes (LexisNexis online) (amended in August 2005 but
    new version was unavailable)
        Kan. Admin. Regs. §§ 28-1-4, -70-1 to -3 (LexisNexis 2006)

Kentucky
    Statutes (Baldwin's Kentucky Revised Statutes Annotated)
        Ky. Rev. Stat. Ann. § 214.556 (West 2005)
    Administrative Codes (Kentucky Administrative Regulation Service)
        None

Louisiana
    Statutes (West's Louisiana Revised Statutes Annotated)
        La. Rev. Stat. Ann. § 40:41 (West Supp. 2006)
        La. Rev. Stat. Ann. § 40:1299.80 to -.87 (West Supp. 2006)
        La. Rev. Stat. Ann. § 44:7 (West Supp. 2006)
    Administrative Codes (Weil's Louisiana Administrative Code)
        La. Code R. tit. 51, §§ II.101-09 (Weil 2004)

Maine
    Statutes (Maine Revised Statutes Annotated [West])
        Me. Rev. Stat. Ann. tit. 22, §§ 1401–1407 (2004 and Supp. 2005)
    Administrative Codes (Code of Main Rules [Weil])
        10-144-253 Me. Code R. § 5 (Weil 1999)
        10-144-255 Me. Code R. §§ 1–6 (Weil 1996)

Maryland
    Statutes (West's Annotated Code of Maryland)
        Md. Code Ann., Health-Gen. §§ 13-1101 to -1116 (West 2005)
        Md. Code Ann., Health-Gen. §§ 18-203 to -204 (West 2005)
    Administrative Codes (Code of Maryland Regulations)
        Md. Code Regs. 10.14.01.01 to -.06 (2003)

Massachusetts
    Statutes (Code of Massachusetts Regulations)
        Mass. Gen. Laws Ann. ch. 111, § 111B (Supp. 2006)
    Administrative Codes (Code of Massachusetts Regulations)
        105 Mass. Code Regs. 301.001 to -.040 (2004)

Michigan
    Statutes (Michigan Compiled Laws Annotated (West)
        Mich. Comp. Laws. § 333.2618 , to -.2619, -.2621, -.2623 (2005)
    Administrative Codes (Michigan Administrative Code, Conway Greene,
    LexisNexis)
        Mich. Admin. Code R. 325.971 (1999)
        Mich. Admin. Code R. 325-9050 to -9057 (LexisNexis 2006)

Minnesota
   Statutes (Minnesota Statutes)
      Minn. Stat. §§ 144.671-69 (2004)
   Administrative Codes (Minnesota Rules)
      Minn. R. 4606.3300 to -.3309 (2005)

Mississippi
   Statutes (Mississippi Code 1972 Annotated [LexisNexis])
      Miss. Code Ann. § 41-91-1 to -15 (2004)
   Administrative Codes (Code of Mississippi Rules [Weil])
      None found

Missouri
   Statutes (Missouri Revised Statutes)
      Mo. Rev. Stat. §§ 192.650 to -657 (2000)
   Administrative Codes (Missouri Code of State Regulations Annotated)
      Mo. Code Regs. Ann. tit. 19, § 70-21-.010 (2000)

Montana
   Statutes (Montana Code Annotated)
      Mont. Code Ann. §§ 50-15-701 to -710 (2005)
      Mont. Code Ann. § 50-16-525 (2005)
   Administrative Codes (Administrative Rules of Montana)
      Mont. Admin. R. 37.8.1801–1808 (2003)

Nebraska
   Statutes (Revised Statutes of Nebraska)
      Neb. Rev. Stat. § 81-638 to -650 (2003)
   Administrative Codes (Nebraska Administrative Codes)
      174 Neb. Admin. Code §§ 5-001 to -011 (2003)
      186 Neb. Admin. Code §§ 1-001 to -009 (2003)

Nevada
   Statutes (Nevada Revised Statutes)
      Nev. Rev. Stat. §§ 457.230 to -280 (2004)
   Administrative Codes (Nevada Administrative Codes)
      Nev. Admin. Code §§ 457.010 to -.150 (2004)

New Hampshire
   Statutes (New Hampshire Revised Statutes Annotated (West)
      N.H. Rev. Stat. Ann. § 141-b:5-10 (2005)
   Administrative Codes (Code of New Hampshire Rules [Weil])
      N.H. Code R. He-P 304.01 to -.07 (Weil 2005)

New Jersey
   Statutes (New Jersey Statutes Annotated [West])
      N.J. Stat. Ann. § 26:1-104 to -108 (1996 and Supp. 2006)
   Administrative Codes (New Jersey Administrative Code [West])
      N. J. Admin. Code § 8:57A-1.1 to -.14 (Supp. 2005)

New Mexico
   Statutes (New Mexico Statutes 1978)
      None found

Administrative Codes (Code of New Mexico Rules [Weil])
N.M. Code R. § 7.4.3.1 to -.13 (Weil 2003)

New York

Statutes (New York Consolidated Law Service [LexisNexis])
N.Y. Pub. Health Law § 2401–2403 (Consol. 2002)

Administrative Codes (Official Compilation of Codes, Rules and Regulations of the State of New York [West])
N. Y. Comp. Codes R. and Regs. tit. 10, § 1.30 to .31 (1995)

North Carolina

Statutes (General Statutes of North Carolina)
N.C. Gen. Stat. §§ 130A-205 to -215 (2005)

Administrative Codes (North Carolina Administrative Codes [West])
10A N.C. Admin. Code 47A.0101 to -.0109 (2004)

North Dakota

Statutes (North Dakota Century Code [LexisNexis])
N.D. Cent. Code § 23-07-01 (Supp. 2005)

Administrative Codes (North Dakota Administrative Code)
N.D. Admin. Code 33-06-01-01 (2004)

Ohio

Statutes (Page's Ohio Revised Code Annotated [LexisNexis])
Ohio Rev. Code Ann. § 3701.261 to -.264 (LexisNexis 2005)

Administrative Codes (Baldwin's Ohio Administrative Code [West])
Ohio Admin. Code 3701:4-1 to -3 (2002)

Oklahoma

Statutes (Oklahoma Statutes [West])
Okla. Stat. tit. 63 § 1-522 (2004)
Okla. Stat. tit. 63 § 1-551.1 (2004)

Administrative Codes (Oklahoma Administrative Code)
Okla. Admin. Code §§ 310:567-1-1 to -2 (2001)
Okla. Admin. Code §§ 310:567-3-1 to -3 (2001)
Okla. Admin. Code §§ 310:567-5-1 to -4 (2001)

Oregon

Statutes (Oregon Revised Statutes)
Or. Rev. Stat. § 432.500-570 (2005)

Administrative Codes (Oregon Administrative Rules)
Or. Admin. R. 333-010-0000 to -0090 (2006)
Or. Admin. R. 410-014-0000 (2006)

Pennsylvania

Statutes (Pennsylvania Consolidated Statutes Annotated)
35 Pa. Cons. Stat. Ann. §§ 5633–5634 (West 2003)
35 Pa. Cons. Stat. Ann. § 5636 (West 2003)
35 Pa. Cons. Stat. Ann. §§ 521.1 to -.5 (West 2003 and Supp. 2006)
35 Pa. Cons. Stat. Ann. §§ 521.15 (West 2003 and Supp. 2006)

Administrative Codes (Pennsylvania Code)
28 Pa. Code § 27.1 to -.31 (2002)

Rhode Island
    Statutes (General Laws of Rhode Island)
        R.I. Gen. Laws § 5-37.3 to -.4 (2004) (amended by 2006) R.I.
            Pub. Laws__available at www.rilin.state.ri.us/PublicLaws/law06/
            law06216 (minimal changes to the section numbers)
        R.I. Gen. Laws § 23-12-4 (2001)
    Administrative Codes (Code of Rhode Island Rules)
        R.I. Code R. 14 000 003 § 1-9 (2002)

South Carolina
    Statutes (Code of Laws of South Carolina)
        S.C.CodeAnn.§30-4-40(1991andSupp.2005)(amendedby2006)S.C.Acts
            __ available at www.scstatehouse.net/sess116_2005-2006/bilss/4456
        S.C. Code Ann. § 44-1-110 (2002 and Supp. 2005)
        S.C. Code Ann. §§ 44-35-10 to -100 (2002)
    Administrative Codes (South Carolina Code of Regulations)
        S.C. Code Ann. Regs. R 61-45A-H (Supp. 2005)

South Dakota
    Statutes (South Dakota Codified Laws)
        S.D. Codified Laws §§ 1-43-11 to -18 (Michie 2004 and Supp. 2006)
        S.D. Codified Laws § 34-14-1 (Michie 2004)
    Administrative Codes (Administrative Rules of South Dakota)
        S.D. Admin. R. 44:22:01:01–03 (2005)
        S.D. Admin. R. 44:22:02:01–10 (2005)
        S.D. Admin. R. 44:22:03:01–03 (2005)
        S.D. Admin. R. 44:22:04:01–03 (2005)
        S.D. Admin. R. 44:22:05:01 (2005)

Tennessee
    Statutes (Tennessee Code Annotated)
        Tenn. Code Ann. §§ 68-1-1001 to -1011 (2001)
    Administrative Codes (Rules and Regulations of the State of Tennessee)
        Tenn. Comp. R. and Regs. 1200-7-2-.01 to -.08 (2002)

Texas
    Statutes (Texas Statutes Annotated)
        Tex. Health and Safety Code Ann. §§ 82.001 to -.011 (Vernon's
            Supp. 2006)
    Administrative Codes (Texas Administrative Code)
        25 Tex. Admin. Code §§ 91.1 to -.12 (2006)

Utah
    Statutes (Utah Code Annotated)
        Utah Code Ann. § 26-1-30 (1998 and Supp. 2006)
        Utah Code Ann. § 26-5-2 to -3 (1998 and Supp. 2006)
        Utah Code Ann. § 26-3-1 to -11 (1998 and Supp. 2006)
    Administrative Codes (Utah Administrative Code)
        Utah Admin. Code r. 384-100-1 to -10 (2006)

Vermont
    Statutes (Vermont Statutes Annotated)
        Vt. Stat. Ann. Tit. 18, §§ 151–157 (2002)
    Administrative Codes (Code of Vermont Rules)
        Vt. Code. R. 13 140 052 §§ 1–3 (2004)
Virginia
    Statutes (Code of Virginia Annotated)
        Va. Code Ann. §§ 32.1-70 to -70.2 (Michie 2004)
        Va. Code Ann. §§ 32.1-71 to -71.2 (Michie 2004)
    Administrative Codes (Virginia Administrative Code)
        12 Va. Admin. Code §§ 5-90-10 (West 2005)
        12 Va. Admin. Code §§ 5-90-150 to -180 (West 2005)
Washington
    Statutes (Revised Code of Washington)
        Wash. Rev. Code §§ 70.54.220 to -270 (2006)
    Administrative Codes (Washington Administrative Code)
        Wash. Admin. Code § 246-101-230 (2005)
        Wash. Admin. Code § 246-101-301 to -320 (2005)
        Wash. Admin. Code § 246-102-001 to -070 (2005)
West Virginia
    Statutes (West Virginia Code Annotated)
        W. Va. Code Ann. § 16-5A-1 to -2a (LexisNexis 2001 and Supp. 2006)
    Administrative Codes (West Virginia Code of State Rules)
        W. Va. Code St. R. § 64-68-1 to -7 (2006)
Wisconsin
    Statutes (Wisconsin Statutes Annotated)
        Wis. Stat. Ann. §§ 255.02 to .04 (West 2004)
    Administrative Codes (Wisconsin Administrative Code)
        Wis. Admin. Code HFS § 124.05 (2006)
Wyoming
    Statutes (Wyoming Statutes Annotated)
        Wyo. Stat. Ann § 35-1-240 (2005)
        Wyo. Stat. Ann § 35-2-609 (2005) amended by 2006 Wyo. Sess. Laws 114
    Administrative Codes (Wyoming Administrative Code)
        048-144-001 Wyo. Code R. §§ 1–7 (Weil 1998)
        048-144-002 Wyo. Code R. §§ 1–6 (Weil 1998)
        048-144-003 Wyo. Code R. § 1 (Weil 1998)

Author Index

Subject Index

Milton Keynes UK
Ingram Content Group UK Ltd.
UKHW040106071024
449327UK00019B/842